D0000658

AN INTRODUCTION

Epidemiology

AN INTRODUCTION

KENNETH J. ROTHMAN

OXFORD
UNIVERSITY PRESS
2002

OXFORD
UNIVERSITY PRESS

Oxford   New York
Athens   Auckland   Bangkok   Bogotá   Buenos Aires   Cape Town
Chennai   Dar es Salaam   Delhi   Florence   Hong Kong   Istanbul   Karachi
Kolkata   Kuala Lumpur   Madrid   Melbourne   Mexico City   Mumbai   Nairobi
Paris   São Paulo   Shanghai   Singapore   Taipei   Tokyo   Toronto   Warsaw

and associated companies in
Berlin   Ibadan

Copyright © 2002 by Oxford University Press, Inc.

Published by Oxford University Press Inc.,
198 Madison Avenue, New York, New York 10016

Oxford is a registered trademark of Oxford University Press.

Library of Congress Cataloging-in-Publication Data
Rothman, Kenneth J.
Epidemiology : an introduction / Kenneth J. Rothman.
p. ; cm.
Includes bibliographical references and index.
ISBN 0-19-513553-9 (C : alk. paper) — ISBN 0-19-513554-7 (P)
1. Epidemiology. I. Title.
[DNLM: 1. Epidemiology. 2. Epidemiologic Methods.
WA 105 R846ea 2002]   RA651 .R68 2002   614.4—dc21   2001036737

7 8 9

Printed in the United States of America
on acid-free paper.

To Emily, Margaret, and Samantha

Preface

Some observers of epidemiology appear to believe that epidemiology is little more than the application of statistical methods to the problems of disease occurrence and causation. In reality, epidemiology is much more than finely dressed statistics. It is a scientific discipline with roots in biology, logic, and the philosophy of science. For epidemiologists, statistical methods serve as an important tool, but not as a foundation. My aim in this book is to present a simple overview of the concepts that are the underpinnings of epidemiology, so that a coherent picture of epidemiologic thinking emerges for the student. The emphasis is not on statistics, formulas, or computation, but on epidemiologic principles and concepts.

For some, epidemiology is too simple to warrant serious attention, and for others it is too convoluted to understand. I hope to demonstrate to the reader that neither view is correct. The first chapter illustrates that epidemiology is more than just applying "common sense," unless one has uncommonly good common sense. Although it is unusual to begin an epidemiology text with a discussion of confounding, I believe that the problem of confounding exemplifies why we need epidemiologic discipline to prevent our inferences from going astray. At the other extreme, those who believe that epidemiology is too complicated might think differently if they had a unifying set of ideas that extend across the boundaries of the many separate topics within epidemiology. My goal in this book has been to provide that unifying set of ideas.

These ideas begin with causation and causal inference, which are presented in Chapter 2. All too often these concepts are skipped over in scientific education. Nevertheless, for epidemiologists they are bedrock concerns that belong in any introduction to the field. Chapter 3 continues with a description of the basic epidemiologic measures, and Chapter 4 covers the main study types. An important thread for the student is the emphasis on measurement, and how to reduce or describe measurement error. Chapters 5 and 6 deal with measurement error. Systematic error, or bias, is treated first, in Chapter 5, and random error in Chapter 6. Chapter 7 introduces the basic analytic methods for estimating epidemiologic effects; these methods are extended in Chapter 8 to stratified data. Chapters 9 and 10 address the more advanced topics of interaction and multivariable modeling. These are subjects to be explored in more advanced courses, but their presentation here in elementary terms lays the groundwork for advanced study. It also draws a boundary between the epidemiologic approach to these topics and non-epidemiologic approaches that steer the analysis in the wrong direction. The final chapter deals with clinical epidemiology, a branch that is growing in scope and importance.

These topics are intended to constitute the core of a first course in epidemiology. Many epidemiology teachers will find that some subjects that they might like to include in such a course, such as the history of epidemiology, the study of infectious illness, or the social determinants of health and disease, have been omitted. To include these and other topics, however, would have made this a different book than the one I set out to write. My intent was not to create a comprehensive survey of the field, but rather a lean text that focuses on key conceptual issues.

Epidemiologic concepts are evolving, as any comparison of this text with earlier books will reveal. To complement the book, the publisher has graciously agreed to host a web site that will support reader participation in discussing, extending and revising points presented in the book. To begin, the web site will post contributed answers to the questions raised at the end of each chapter in the text. Interested readers can find the web site at http://www.oup-usa.org/epi/rothman.

Along the way I have received invaluable feedback from many students and colleagues. I am especially grateful to Kristin Anderson, Georgette Baghdady, Dan Brooks, Bob Green, Sander Greenland, Bettie Nelson, Ya-Fen Purvis, Igor Schillevoort, Bahi Takkouche, and Noel Weiss. Cristina Cann provided unflagging and generous encouragement. Katarina Augustsson deserves special mention for her careful reading of the manuscript and patient helpful criticisms. Finally, I am indebted to my colleague Janet Lang, who gently prodded me at the right time and was an inspiration throughout.

Contents

Epidemiology
AN INTRODUCTION

1

Introduction to
Epidemiologic Thinking

This book presents the basic concepts and methods of epidemiology. Often considered the core science of public health, epidemiology involves "the study of the distribution and determinants of disease frequency"[1] or, put even more simply, "the study of the occurrence of illness."[2]

The principles of epidemiologic research appear deceptively simple, which misleads some people into believing that anyone can master epidemiology just by applying common sense. The problem with this view is that the kind of common sense that is required may be elusive without training in epidemiologic concepts and methods. In this chapter, we glimpse some examples of the epidemiologic concept of confounding as a way to introduce epidemiologic thinking.

Common sense tells us that residents of Sweden, where the standard of living is generally high, should have lower death rates than residents of Panama, where poverty and more limited health care take their toll. Surprisingly, however, a greater proportion of Swedish residents than Panamanian residents die each year. This fact belies common sense. The explanation lies in the age distributions of the populations of Sweden and Panama. Figure 1–1 shows the population pyramids of the two countries. A *population pyramid* displays the age distribution of a population graphically. The population pyramid for Panama tapers dramatically from younger to older age groups, reflecting the fact that most Panamanians are in the younger age categories. In contrast, the population pyramid of Sweden is more rectangular, with roughly the same number of people in each of the age categories up to about age 60 and some tapering above that age. As these graphs make clear, Swedes tend to be older than Panamanians. For people of the same age in the two countries, the death rate among Swedes is indeed lower than that of Panamanians, but in both places older people die at a greater rate than younger people. Because Sweden has a population that is on the average older than that of Panama, a greater proportion of all Swedes die in

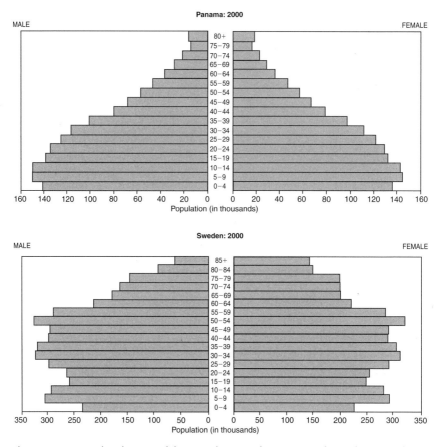

Figure 1–1. Age distribution of the populations of Panama and Sweden (population pyramids). Source: U.S. Census Bureau, International Data Base.

a given year, despite the lower death rates within age categories in Sweden compared with Panama.

This situation illustrates what epidemiologists call *confounding.* In this example, age differences between the countries are confounding the differences in death rates. Confounding occurs commonly in epidemiologic comparisons. Consider the following mortality data, summarized from a study that looked at smoking habits of residents of Whickham, England, in the period 1972–1974 and then tracked the survival over the next 20 years of those who were interviewed.[3–5] Among 1314 women in the survey, nearly half were smokers. Oddly, proportionately fewer of the smokers died during the ensuing 20 years than nonsmokers. The data are reproduced in Table 1–1.

Only 24% of the women who were smokers at the time of the initial survey died during the 20-year follow-up period. In contrast, 31% of those who were nonsmokers died during the follow-up period. Does

Table 1–1. Risk of death in a 20-year period among women in Whickham, England, according to their smoking status at the beginning of the period*

Vital Status	Smoker	Nonsmoker	Total
Dead	139	230	369
Alive	443	502	945
Total	582	732	1314
Risk (dead/total)	0.24	0.31	0.28

*Data from Vanderpump et al.[5]

this difference indicate that women who were smokers fared better than women who were not smokers? Not necessarily. One difficulty that many readers quickly spot is that the smoking information was obtained only once, at the start of the follow-up period. Smoking habits for some women will have changed during the follow-up. Could those changes explain the results that appear to confer an advantage on the smokers? It is theoretically possible that all or many of the smokers quit soon after the survey and that many of the nonsmokers started smoking. While possible, this scenario is implausible, and without evidence for these changes in smoking behavior, this implausible scenario is not a reasonable criticism of the study findings. A more realistic explanation for the unusual finding becomes clear if we examine the data within age categories, as shown in Table 1–2 (the risks for each age group were calculated by dividing the number who died in each smoking group by the total of those dead or alive).

Table 1–1 combines all of the age categories listed in Table 1–2 into a single table, which is called the *crude* data. The more detailed display of the same data in Table 1–2 is called an *age-specific* display, or a display *stratified* by age. The age-specific data show that in the youngest and oldest age categories there was little difference between smokers and nonsmokers in risk of death. Few died among those in the younger age categories, regardless of whether they were smokers or not, whereas among the oldest women, nearly everyone died during the 20 years of follow-up. For women in the middle age categories, however, there was a consistently greater risk of death among smokers than nonsmokers, a pattern contrary to the impression gained from the crude data in Table 1–1.

Why did the nonsmokers have a higher risk of death in the study population as a whole? The reason is evident in Table 1–2: a much greater proportion of the nonsmoking women were in the highest age categories, the age categories that contributed a proportionately greater number of deaths. The difference in the age distributions between smokers and nonsmokers reflects the fact that, for most people, lifelong smoking habits are determined early in life. During the decades preced-

Table 1–2. Risk of death in a 20-year period among women in Whickham, England, according to their smoking status at the beginning of the period, by age*

Age (years)	Vital Status	Smoker	Nonsmoker	Total
	Dead	2	1	3
18–24	Alive	53	61	114
	Risk	0.04	0.02	0.03
	Dead	3	5	8
25–34	Alive	121	152	273
	Risk	0.02	0.03	0.03
	Dead	14	7	21
35–44	Alive	95	114	209
	Risk	0.13	0.06	0.09
	Dead	27	12	39
45–54	Alive	103	66	169
	Risk	0.21	0.15	0.19
	Dead	51	40	91
55–64	Alive	64	81	145
	Risk	0.44	0.33	0.39
	Dead	29	101	130
65–74	Alive	7	28	35
	Risk	0.81	0.78	0.79
	Dead	13	64	77
75+	Alive	0	0	0
	Risk	1.00	1.00	1.00

*Data from Vanderpump et al.[5]

ing the study in Whickham, there was a trend for increasing proportions of young women to become smokers. The oldest women in the Whickham study grew up during a period when few women became smokers, and they tended to remain nonsmokers for the duration of their lives. As time went by, a greater proportion of women who were passing through their teenage or young adult years became smokers. The result is a strikingly different age distribution for the female smokers and non-smokers of Whickham. Were this difference in the age distribution ignored, one might conclude erroneously that smoking was not related to a higher risk of death. In fact, smoking *is* related to a higher risk of death, but confounding by age has obscured this relation in the crude data of Table 1–1. In Chapter 8, we return to these data and show how to calculate the effect of smoking on the risk of death after removing the age confounding.

Confounding is a problem that pervades many epidemiologic studies, but it is by no means the only issue that bedevils epidemiologic inferences. One day, readers of the *Boston Globe,* a local newspaper, opened the paper to find a feature story about orchestra conductors. The point of the article was that conducting an orchestra was salubrious, as evinced by the fact that so many well-known orchestra conductors lived to be extremely old. Common sense suggests that if the people in an occupation tend to live long lives, the occupation must be good for health. Unfortunately, what appeared to be common sense for the author of the article is not very sensible from an epidemiologic point of view. The long-lived conductors cited in the article were mentioned because they lived to be old. Citing selected examples in this way constitutes *anecdotal* information, which can be extremely misleading. For all we know, the reporter searched specifically for examples of elderly conductors and overlooked other conductors who might have died at an earlier age. Most epidemiologists would not classify anecdotal information as epidemiologic data at all.

Furthermore, the reporter's observation has problems that go beyond the reliance on anecdotes instead of a formal evaluation. Suppose that the reporter had identified all orchestra conductors who worked in the United States during the past 100 years and studied their longevity. This approach would avoid relying on hand-picked examples, but it still suffers from an important problem that would lead to an incorrect answer. The problem is that orchestra conductors are not born as orchestra conductors. They become conductors at a point in their careers when they may have already attained a respectable age. If we start with a group of people who are 40 years old, on the average they are likely to survive to an older age than the typical person who was just born. Why? Because they have a 40-year head start; if they died before age 40, they could not be part of a group in which everyone is 40 years old. To find out if conducting an orchestra is beneficial to health, we should compare the risk of death among orchestra conductors with the risk of death among other people who have attained the same age as the conductors. Simply noting the average age at death of the conductors will give the wrong answer, even if all orchestra conductors were to be studied.

Here is another example that makes this point clearly. Suppose that we study two groups of people and look at the average age at death among those who die. In group A, the average age at death is 4 years; in group B, it is 28 years. Can we say that being a member of group A is riskier than being a member of group B? We cannot, for the same reason that the age at death of orchestra conductors was misleading. Suppose that group A comprises nursery school students and group B comprises military commandos. It would be no surprise that the average age at death of people who are currently military commandos is 28 years or that the average age at death of people who are currently nursery school students is 4 years. Still, we suspect that being a military commando is riskier than being a nursery school student and that these data on the average age at death do not address the issue of which of these groups faces a greater risk of death. When one looks at the average age at death, one looks only at those who actually die and ignores all those who survive. Consequently, average age at death does not reflect the risk of death but only a characteristic of those who die.

In a study of factory workers, an investigator inferred that the factory work was dangerous because the average age at onset of a particular kind of cancer was lower in these workers than among the general population. But just as for the nursery school students and the military commandos, if these workers were young, the cancers that occurred among them would have to be occurring in young people. Furthermore, the age at onset of a disease does not take into account what proportion of people get the disease.

These examples reflect the fallacy of comparing the average age at which death or disease strikes rather than comparing the risk of death between groups of the same age. We will explore the proper way to make epidemiologic comparisons in later chapters. The point of these examples is to illustrate that a common-sense approach to a simple problem can be overtly wrong, until we educate our common sense to appreciate better the nature of the problem. Any sensible person can understand epidemiology, but without considering the principles outlined in this book, even a sensible person using very common sense is apt to go astray. By mastering a few fundamental epidemiologic principles, it is possible to refine our common sense to avoid these traps.

Questions

1. Age is a variable that is often responsible for confounding in epidemiology, in part because the occurrence of many diseases changes with age. The change in disease risk with age is often referred to as the effect of age. Does it make sense to think of age as having an effect on disease risk, or is it more sensible to think that the effect of age is itself confounded by other factors?

2. More people in Los Angeles die from cardiovascular disease each year than do people in San Francisco. What is the most important explanation for this difference? What additional factors would you consider to explain the difference in the number of deaths?

3. In Table 1–2, which age group would you say shows the greatest effect of smoking on the risk of death during the 20-year interval? How have you defined "greatest effect"? What other way could you have defined it? Does your answer depend on which definition you use?

4. On a piece of graph paper, use the data in Table 1–2 to plot the 20-year risk of death against age. Put age on the horizontal axis and the 20-year risk of death on the vertical axis. Describe the shape of the curve. What biologic forces account for the shape?

5. A physician who was interested in jazz studied the age at death of jazz musicians, whom he identified from an encyclopedia of jazz. He found that the average age at death of the jazz musicians was about the same as that of the general population. He concluded that this finding refuted the prevailing wisdom that jazz musicians tended to live dissolute lives and thus experienced greater mortality than other people. Explain his error.

6. A researcher determined that being left-handed was dangerous because he found that the average age at death of left-handers was lower than that of right-handers. Was he correct? Why or why not?

7. What is the underlying problem in comparing the average age at death or the average age at which a person gets a specific disease between two populations? How should you avert this problem?

References

1. MacMahon, B, Pugh, TF: *Epidemiology: Principles and Methods,* Chapter 1, Boston: Little, Brown, 1970.
2. Cole, P: The evolving case-control study. *J Chron Dis* 1979;32:15–27.
3. Appleton, DR, French, JM, Vanderpump, MPJ: Ignoring a covariate: an example of Simpson's paradox. *Am Statistician* 1996;50:340–341.
4. Tunbridge, WMG, Evered, DC, Hall, R, et al.: The spectrum of thyroid disease in a community. *Clin Endocrinol* 1977;7:481–493.
5. Vanderpump, MPJ, Tunbridge, WMG, French, JM, et al: The incidence of thyroid disorders in the community: a twenty-year follow-up of the Whickham survey. *Clin Endocrinol* 1995;43:55–69.

2

What Is Causation?

The acquired wisdom that certain conditions or events bring about other conditions or events is an important survival trait. Consider an infant whose first experiences are a jumble of sensations that include hunger pangs, thirst, color, light, heat, cold, and many other stimuli. Gradually, the infant begins to perceive patterns in the jumble and to anticipate connections between actions such as crying and effects such as being fed. Eventually, the infant assembles an inventory of associated perceptions. We can imagine that the concept slowly develops that some of these phenomena are causally related to others that follow. Along with this growing appreciation for specific causal relations comes the general concept that some events or conditions can be considered causes of other events or conditions.

Thus, our first appreciation of the concept of causation is based on our own observations. These observations typically involve causes with effects that are immediately apparent. For example, when one changes the position of a light switch on the wall, one can see the instant effect of the light going on or off. There is more to the causal mechanism for getting the light to shine than turning the light switch to the "on" position, however. Suppose the electric lines to the building are down in a storm. Turning on the switch will have no effect. Suppose the bulb is burned out. Again, the switch will have no effect. One cause of the light going on is having the switch in the proper place, but along with it we must include a supply of power to the circuit, a working bulb, and wiring. When all other factors are already in place, turning the switch will cause the light to go on, but if one or more of the other factors is not playing its causal role, the light will not go on when the switch is turned. There is a tendency to consider the switch to be the unique cause of turning on the light, but in reality we can define a more intricate causal mechanism, in which the switch is one component of several. The tendency to identify the switch as the unique cause stems from its usual role as the final factor that acts in the causal mechanism. The wiring can be considered part of the causal mechanism, but once it is put in place, it seldom warrants further attention. The switch, however, is often the only part of the mechanism that needs to be activated to obtain the effect of turning on the light. The effect usually occurs immediately after turning the switch, and as a result we slip into a frame of thinking in which we identify the switch as a unique cause. The inadequacy of this assumption is emphasized when the bulb goes bad and needs to be replaced.

The Causal Pie Model

Causes of disease can be conceptualized in the same way as the causes of turning on a light. A helpful way to think about causal mechanisms of disease is depicted in Figure 2–1.[1] Each "pie" in the diagram represents a theoretical *causal mechanism* for a given disease, sometimes called a "sufficient cause." There are three pies, to illustrate that there are multiple mechanisms that cause any type of disease. Each individual instance of disease will occur through a single mechanism or sufficient cause. A given causal mechanism requires the joint action of many component factors, or *component causes.* Each component cause is an event or condition that plays a necessary role in the occurrence of some cases of a given disease. For example, the disease might be cancer of the lung and, in the first mechanism in Figure 2–1, factor C might be cigarette smoking. The other factors would include genetic traits or other environmental exposures that play a causal role in cancer of the lung. Some component causes would presumably act in many different causal mechanisms.

Implications of the Causal Pie Model

Multicausality

The model of causation showed in Figure 2–1 illuminates several important principles regarding causes. Perhaps the most important of these principles is self-evident from the model: every causal mechanism in-

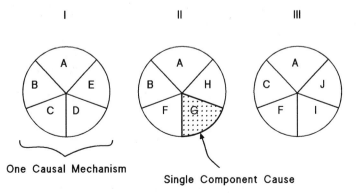

Figure 2–1. Three sufficient causes of a disease.

Genetic versus environmental causes

It is a strong assertion that every case of every disease has both genetic and environmental causes. Nevertheless, if all genetic factors that determine disease are taken into account, then essentially 100% of disease can be said to be inherited, in the sense that nearly all cases of disease have some genetic component causes. What would be the genetic component causes of someone who gets drunk and is killed in an automobile after colliding with a tree? It is easy to conceive of genetic traits that lead to psychiatric problems such as alcoholism, which in turn lead to drunk driving and consequent fatality. Analogously, one can also claim that essentially 100% of any disease is environmentally caused, even those diseases that we often consider to be purely genetic. Phenylketonuria, for example, is considered by many to be purely genetic. Nonetheless, if we consider the disease that phenylketonuria represents to be the mental retardation that may result from it, we can prevent the disease by appropriate dietary intervention. Thus, we can say that the disease has environmental determinants. Although it may seem like an exaggeration to claim that 100% of any disease is environmental and genetic at the same time, it is a good approximation. It may seem counterintuitive because most of the time we cannot manipulate many of the causes and the ones that can be controlled tend to be either environmental or genetic but usually not both.

volves the joint action of a multitude of component causes. Consider as an example the cause of a broken hip. Suppose that someone experiences a traumatic injury to the head that leads to a permanent disturbance in equilibrium. Many years later, the faulty equilibrium plays a causal role in a fall that occurs while the person is walking on an icy path. The fall results in a broken hip. Other factors playing a causal role for the broken hip could include the type of shoe the person was wearing, the lack of a handrail along the path, a strong wind, and the weight of the person. The complete causal mechanism involves a multitude of factors. Some factors, such as the earlier injury that resulted in the equilibrium disturbance and the weight of the person, reflect earlier events that have had a lingering effect. Some causal components of the broken hip are genetic. Genetic factors would affect the person's weight, gait, behavior, and recovery from the earlier trauma. Other factors, such as the force of the wind, are clearly environmental. It is reasonably safe to assert that there are nearly always some genetic and some environmental component causes in every causal mechanism. (Here, we use *environmental* to mean simply nongenetic.) Apparently, even an event such as a fall on an icy path leading to a broken hip is part of a complicated causal mechanism that involves many component causes.

Strength of Causes

It is common to think that some component causes play a more important role than others in the causation of disease. One way this concept is
expressed is by the strength of a causal effect. Thus, we say that smoking has a strong effect on lung cancer risk because smokers have about
10 times the risk of lung cancer as nonsmokers. On the other hand, we
say that smoking has a weaker effect on myocardial infarction because
the risk of a heart attack is only about twice as great in smokers as in
nonsmokers. With respect to an individual case of disease, however,
every component cause that played a role in bringing that case into existence was necessary to the occurrence of that case. According to the
causal pie model, for a given case of disease, there is no such thing as a
strong cause or a weak cause. There is only a distinction between factors
that were causes and factors that were not causes.

To understand what epidemiologists mean by *strength* of a cause, we
need to shift from thinking about an individual case to thinking about
the total burden of cases occurring in a population. We can then define a
strong cause to be a component cause that plays a causal role in a large
proportion of cases, whereas a weak cause would be a causal component in a small proportion of cases. Because smoking plays a causal role
in a high proportion of the lung cancer cases, we call it a strong cause of
lung cancer. For a given case of lung cancer, smoking is no more important than any of the other component causes for that case; but on the
population level, it is considered a strong cause of lung cancer because it
causes such a large proportion of cases.

The strength of a cause, defined in this way, necessarily depends on
the prevalence of other causal factors that produce disease. As a result,
the concept of a strong or weak cause cannot be a universally accurate
description of any cause. For example, suppose we say that smoking is a
strong cause of lung cancer because it plays a causal role in a large
proportion of cases. Exposure to ambient radon gas, in contrast, is a
weaker cause because it has a causal role in a much smaller proportion
of lung cancer cases. Now imagine that society eventually succeeds in
eliminating tobacco smoking, with a consequent reduction in smoking-
related cases of lung cancer. One result is that a much larger proportion of
the lung cancer cases that continue to occur will be caused by exposure to
radon gas. It would appear that eliminating smoking has strengthened
the causal effect of radon gas on lung cancer. This example illustrates
that what we mean by strength of effect is not a biologically stable characteristic of a factor. From the biologic perspective, the causal role of a
factor in producing disease is neither strong nor weak: the biology of
causation corresponds simply to the identity of the component causes in
a causal mechanism. The proportion of the population burden of disease
that a factor causes, which we use to define the strength of a cause, can
change from population to population and over time if there are changes

in the distribution of other causes of the disease. In short, the strength of a cause does not equate with the biology of causation.

Interaction between Causes

The causal pie model posits that several causal components act in concert to produce an effect. "Acting in concert" does not necessarily imply that factors must act at the same time. Consider the example above of the person who sustained trauma to the head that resulted in an equilibrium disturbance, which led years later to a fall on an icy path. The earlier head trauma played a causal role in the later hip fracture, as did the weather conditions on the day of the fracture. If both of these factors played a causal role in the hip fracture, then they interacted with one another to cause the fracture, despite the fact that their time of action was many years apart. We would say that any and all of the factors in the same causal mechanism for disease interact with one another to cause disease. Thus, the head trauma interacted with the weather conditions as well as with the other component causes, such as the type of footwear, the absence of a handhold, and any other conditions that were necessary to the causal mechanism of the fall and the broken hip that resulted. One can view each causal pie as a set of interacting causal components. This model provides a biologic basis for the concept of interaction that differs from the more traditional statistical view of interaction. We discuss the implication of this difference later, in Chapter 9.

Sum of Attributable Fractions

Consider the data in Table 2–1, which shows the rate of head-and-neck cancer according to smoking status and alcohol exposure. Suppose that the differences in the rates reflect causal effects. Among those who are smokers and alcohol drinkers, what proportion of cases of head and neck cancer that occur is attributable to the effect of smoking? We know that the rate for these people is 12 cases per 10,000 person-years. If these same people were not smokers, we can infer that their rate of head-and-neck cancer would be 3 cases per 10,000 person-years. If this difference reflects the causal role of smoking, then we might infer that 9 out of every 12 cases, or 75%, are attributable to smoking among those who smoke and drink alcohol. If we turn the question around and ask what proportion of disease among these same people is attributable to alcohol drinking, we would attribute 8 out of every 12 cases, or 67%, to alcohol drinking.

Can we attribute 75% of the cases to smoking and 67% to alcohol drinking among those who are exposed to both? The answer is yes, because when we do so, some cases are counted more than once as a result of the interaction between smoking and alcohol. These cases are attributable both to smoking and to alcohol drinking, because both factors played a causal role in producing those cases. One consequence of inter-

Table 2–1. Hypothetical rates of head-and-neck cancer (cases per 10,000 person-years) according to smoking status and alcohol drinking

Smoking Status	Nondrinker	Drinker
Nonsmoker	1	3
Smoker	4	12

action is that we should not expect that the proportions of disease attributable to various component causes will sum to 100%.

A widely discussed but unpublished paper from the 1970s written by scientists at the National Institutes of Health proposed that as much as 40% of cancer is attributable to occupational exposures. Many scientists thought that this fraction was an overestimate and argued against the claim.[2,3] One of the arguments used in rebuttal was as follows: x% of cancer is caused by smoking, y% by diet, z% by alcohol, and so on; when all of these percentages are added up, only a small percentage, much less than 40, is left for occupational causes. But this rebuttal is fallacious because it is based on the naive view that every case of disease has a single cause and that two causes cannot contribute to the same case of cancer. In fact, since diet, smoking, asbestos, and various occupational exposures, along with other factors, interact with one another and with genetic factors to cause cancer, each case of cancer could be attributed repeatedly to many separate component causes. The sum of disease attributable to various component causes in reality has no upper limit.

Induction Time

Because the component causes in a given causal mechanism do not act simultaneously, there will usually be a period of time between the action of a component cause and the completion of a sufficient cause. The only exception is the last component cause to act in a given causal mechanism. The last-acting component cause completes the causal mechanism, and we can say that disease begins concurrently with its action. For earlier-acting component causes, we can define the *induction period* as the period of time beginning at the action of a component cause and ending when the final component cause acts and the disease occurs. For example, in our illustration of the fractured hip, the induction time between the head trauma that resulted in an equilibrium disturbance and the later hip fracture was many years. The induction time between the decision to wear nongripping shoes and the hip fracture may have been a matter of minutes or hours. The induction time between the gust of wind that triggered the fall and the hip fracture might have been seconds or less.

In an individual instance, we would not be able to learn the exact length of an induction period, since we cannot be sure of the causal mechanism that produces disease in an individual instance or when all of the relevant component causes in that mechanism acted. With research data, however, we can learn enough to characterize the induction period that relates the action of a single component cause to the occurrence of disease in general. A clear example of a lengthy induction time is the cause–effect relation between exposure of a female fetus to diethylstilbestrol (DES) and the subsequent development of adenocarcinoma of the vagina. The cancer is usually diagnosed between the ages of 15 and 30 years. Since the causal exposure to DES occurs during gestation, there is an induction time of about 15 to 30 years for its carcinogenic action. During this time, other causes presumably operate; some evidence suggests that hormonal action during adolescence may be part of the mechanism.[4]

The causal pie model makes it clear that it is incorrect to characterize a disease itself as having a lengthy or brief induction time. The induction time can be conceptualized only in relation to a specific component cause. Thus, we say that the induction time relating DES exposure to clear cell carcinoma of the vagina is 15 to 30 years, but we cannot say that 15 to 30 years is the induction time for clear cell carcinoma in general. Since each component cause in any causal mechanism can act at a time different from the other component causes, each will have its own induction time. For the component cause that acts last, the induction time always equals 0. If another component cause of clear cell carcinoma of the vagina that acts during adolescence were identified, it would have a much shorter induction time than DES. Thus, induction time characterizes a specific cause–effect pair rather than just the effect.

In carcinogenesis, the terms *initiator* and *promotor* are used to refer to component causes of cancer that act early and late, respectively, in the causal mechanism. Cancer itself has often been characterized as a disease process with a long induction time. This characterization is a misconception, however, because any late-acting component in the causal process, such as a promotor, will have a short induction time and, by definition, the induction time will always be 0 for the last component cause to act.

After disease occurs, its presence is not always immediately apparent. If it becomes apparent later, the time interval between disease occurrence and its subsequent detection, whether by medical testing or by the emergence of symptoms, is termed the *latent period*.[5] The length of the latent period can be reduced by improved methods of disease detection. The induction period, however, cannot be reduced by early detection of disease, because there is no disease to detect until after the induction period is over. Practically, it may be difficult to distinguish between the induction period and the latent period, because there may be no way to establish when the disease process began if it is not detected until later. Thus, diseases such as slow-growing cancers may appear to have long induction periods with respect to many causes, in part because they have long latent periods.

Although it is not possible to reduce the induction period proper by earlier detection of disease, it may be possible to observe intermediate stages of a causal mechanism. The increased interest in biomarkers such as DNA adducts is an example of focusing on causes that are more prox-imal to the disease occurrence. Such biomarkers may reflect the effects on the organism of agents that acted at an earlier time.

Is a catalyst a cause?

Some agents may have a causal action by shortening the induction time of other agents. Suppose that exposure to factor A leads to epi-lepsy after an interval of 10 years, on the average. It may be that expo-sure to a drug, B, would shorten this interval to 2 years. Is B acting as a catalyst or as a cause of epilepsy? The answer is both: a catalyst *is* a cause. Without B, the occurrence of epilepsy comes 8 years later than it comes with B, so we can say that B causes the onset of the early epi-lepsy. It is not sufficient to argue that the epilepsy would have oc-curred anyway, so B is not a cause of its occurrence. First, it would not have occurred at that time, and the time of occurrence is considered part of the definition of an event. Second, epilepsy will occur later only if the person survives an additional 8 years, which is not certain. Therefore, agent B determines when the epilepsy occurs and it can determine whether it occurs at all. For this reason, we consider any agent that acts as a catalyst of a causal mechanism, shortening the induction period for other agents, to be a cause. Similarly, any agent that postpones the onset of an event, drawing out the induction period for another agent, we consider to be a preventive. It should not be too surprising to equate postponement with prevention: we routinely use such an equation when we employ the euphemism that we prevent death, which actually can only be postponed. What we prevent is death at a given time, in favor of death at a later time.

The Process of Scientific Inference

Much of epidemiologic research is aimed at uncovering the causes of disease. Now that we have a conceptual model for causes, how do we go about determining whether a given relation is causal? Some scientists refer to checklists for causal inference, and others focus on complicated statistical approaches, but the answer to this question is not to be found either in checklists or in statistical methods. The question itself is tantamount to asking how we apply the scientific method to epidemiologic research. This question leads directly to the philosophy of science, a topic that goes well beyond the scope of this book. Nevertheless, it is worthwhile to summarize two of the major philosophical doctrines that have influenced modern science.

Induction

Since the rise of modern science in the seventeenth century, scientists and philosophers alike have puzzled over the question of how to determine the truth about assertions that deal with the empirical world. From the time of the ancient Greeks, deductive methods have been used to prove the validity of mathematical propositions. These methods enable us to draw airtight conclusions because they are self-contained, starting with a limited set of definitions and axioms and applying rules of logic that guarantee the validity of the method. Empirical science is different, however. Assertions about the real world do not start from arbitrary axioms, and they involve observations on nature that are fallible and incomplete. These stark differences from deductive logic led early modern empiricists, such as Francis Bacon, to promote what they considered a new type of logic, which they called *induction* (not to be confused with the concept of induction period, discussed above). *Induction* was an indirect method used to gain insight into what has been metaphorically described as the fabric of nature.

The method of induction starts with observations on nature. To the extent that the observations fall into a pattern, the observations are said to induce in the mind of the observer a suggestion of a more general statement about nature. The general statement could range from a simple hypothesis to a more profound natural law or natural relation. The statement about nature will be either reinforced by further observations or refuted by contradictory observations. For example, suppose an investigator in New York conducts an experiment to observe the boiling point of water and observes that the water boils at 100°C. The experiment might be repeated many times, each time showing that the water boils at about 100°C. By induction, the investigator could conclude that the boiling point of water is 100°C. The induction itself involves an inference beyond the observations to a general statement that describes the nature of boiling water. As induction became popular, it was seen to differ considerably from deduction. Although not as well understood as deduction, the approach was considered a new type of logic, inductive logic.

Although induction, with its emphasis on observation, represented an important advance over the appeal to faith and authority that characterized medieval scholasticism, it was not long before the validity of the new logic was questioned. The sharpest criticism came from the philosophical skeptic David Hume, who pointed out that induction had no logical force. Rather, it amounted to an assumption that what had been observed in the past would continue to occur in the future. When supporters of induction argued for the validity of the process because it had been seen to work on numerous occasions, Hume countered that the argument was an example of circular reasoning that relied on induction to justify itself. Hume was so profoundly skeptical that he distrusted any inference based on observation, for the simple reason that observations depend on sense perceptions and are therefore subject to error.

Refutationism

Hume's criticisms of induction have been a powerful force in modern scientific philosophy. Perhaps the most influential reply to Hume was offered by Karl Popper. Popper accepted Hume's point that in empirical science one cannot prove the validity of a statement about nature in any way that is comparable with a deductive proof. Popper's philosophy, known as *refutationism*, held that statements about nature can be corroborated by evidence but that corroboration does not amount to logical proof. On the other hand, Popper asserted that statements about nature can be refuted by deductive logic. To grasp the point, consider the example above regarding the boiling point of water. The refutationist view is that the repeated experiments showing that water boils at 100°C corroborate the hypothesis that water boils at this temperature, but do not prove it.[6] A colleague of the New York researcher who works in Denver, a city at high altitude, might find that water there boils at a much lower temperature. This single contrary observation carries more weight regarding the hypothesis about the boiling point of water than thousands of repetitions of the initial experiment at sea level.

The asymmetrical implications of a refuting observation, on the one hand, and supporting observations, on the other hand, are the essence of the refutationist view. This school of thought encourages scientists to subject a new hypothesis to rigorous tests that might falsify the hypothesis, in preference to repetitions of the initial observations that add little beyond the weak corroboration that replication can supply. The implication for the method of science is that hypotheses should be evaluated by subjecting them to crucial tests. If a test refutes a hypothesis, then a new hypothesis needs to be formulated, which can then be subjected to further tests. Thus, after finding that water boils at a lower temperature in Denver than in New York, one must discard the hypothesis that water boils at 100°C and replace it with a more refined hypothesis, one that will explain the difference in boiling points under different atmospheric pressures. This process describes an endless cycle of *conjecture and refutation*. The conjecture, or hypothesis, is the product of scientific insight and imagination. It requires little justification except that it can account for existing observations. A useful approach is to pose competing hypotheses to explain existing observations and to test them against one another. The refutationist philosophy postulates that all scientific knowledge is tentative in that it may one day need to be refined or even discarded. Under this philosophy, what we call scientific knowledge is a body of as yet unrefuted hypotheses that appear to explain existing observations.

How would an epidemiologist apply refutationist thinking to his or her work? If causal mechanisms are stated specifically, an epidemiologist can construct crucial tests of competing hypotheses. For example, when toxic shock syndrome was first studied, there were two competing hypotheses about the origin of the toxin. Under one hypothesis, the toxin responsible for the disease was a chemical in the tampon, so women using tampons were exposed to the toxin directly from the tampon. Under the other hypothesis, the tampon acted as a culture medium for staphylococci that produced the toxin. Both hypotheses explained the relation of toxic shock occurrence to tampon use. The two hypotheses, however, led to opposite predictions about the relation between the frequency of changing tampons and the risk of toxic shock. Under the hypothesis of a chemical intoxication, more frequent changing of the tampon would lead to more exposure to the toxin and possible absorption of a greater overall dose. This hypothesis predicted that women who changed tampons more frequently would have a higher risk of toxic shock syndrome than women who changed tampons infrequently. The culture-medium hypothesis predicts that the women who changed tampons frequently would have a lower risk than those who left the tampon in for longer periods, because a short duration of use for each tampon would prevent the staphylococci from multiplying enough to produce a damaging dose of toxin. Thus, epidemiologic research, which showed that infrequent changing of tampons was associated with greater risk of toxic shock, refuted the chemical theory.

Causal Criteria

Earlier, we said that there is no simple checklist that can determine whether an observed relation is causal. Nevertheless, attempts at such checklists have appeared and merit comment here. Most of these lists stem from the canons of inference described by John Stuart Mill.[5] The most widely cited list of causal criteria, originally posed as a list of standards, is attributed to Hill,[7] who adapted them from the U.S. Surgeon General's 1964 report on smoking and health.[8] The "Hill criteria," as they are often described, are listed in Table 2–2, along with some problems relating to each of them.

Although Hill did not propose these criteria as a checklist for evaluating whether a reported association might be interpreted as causal, many others have applied them in that way. Admittedly, the process of causal inference as described above is difficult and uncertain, making the appeal of a simple checklist undeniable. Unfortunately, this checklist, like

Table 2–2. "Causal criteria" of Hill

Criterion	Problems with the criterion
1. Strength	Strength depends on the prevalence of other causes and, thus, is not a biologic characteristic; could be confounded
2. Consistency	Exceptions are understood best with hindsight
3. Specificity	A cause can have many effects
4. Temporality	It may be difficult to establish the temporal sequence between cause and effect
5. Biologic gradient	Could be confounded; threshold phenomena would not show a progressive relation
6. Plausibility	Too subjective
7. Coherence	How does it differ from consistency or plausibility?
8. Experimental evidence	Not always available
9. Analogy	Analogies abound

all others with the same goal, fails to deliver on the hope of clearly distinguishing causal from noncausal relations. Consider the first criterion, strength. It is tempting to believe that strong associations are more likely to be causal than weak ones, but as we have seen above from our discussion of causal pies, not every component cause will have a strong association with the disease that it produces; strength of association depends on the prevalence of other factors. Some causal associations, such as that between cigarette smoking and coronary heart disease, are weak. Furthermore, a strong association could be noncausal, a confounded result stemming from the effect of another risk factor for the disease that is strongly associated with the one under study. For example, birth order is strongly associated with the occurrence of Down syndrome, but it is a confounded association that is completely explained by maternal age. If weak associations can be causal and strong associations can be noncausal, it does not appear that strength of association can be considered a criterion for causality.

The third criterion, specificity, suggests that a relation is more likely to be causal if the exposure is related to a single outcome rather than myriad outcomes. This criterion is misleading: it implies, for example, that the more diseases with which smoking is associated, the greater the evidence that smoking is not causally associated with any of them. Now consider the fifth criterion, biologic gradient. It is often taken as a sign of a causal relation, but it can just as well result from confounding or other biases as from a causal connection. The relation between Down syndrome and birth order mentioned above, for example, shows a biologic gradient despite it being completely explained by confounding from maternal age. Other criteria from Hill's list either are vague (consistency, plausibility, coherence, and analogy) or do not apply in many settings (experimental evidence). The only criterion on the list that is truly a causal criterion is temporality, which implies that the cause comes before the effect. This criterion, which is part of the definition of a cause, is useful to keep in mind, although it may be difficult to establish the proper time sequence for cause and effect. For example, does stress lead to overeating or does overeating lead to stress? In general, it is better to avoid a checklist approach to causal inference and instead to consider approaches such as conjecture and refutation. Checklists lend a deceptive and mindless authority to an inherently imperfect and creative process. In contrast, causal inference based on conjecture and refutation fosters a highly desirable critical scrutiny.

Generalization in Epidemiology

A useful way to think of scientific generalization is to consider a generalization to be the elaboration of a scientific theory. A given study may test the viability of one or more theories. Theories that survive such tests can be viewed as general statements about nature that tell us what to expect in people or settings that were not studied. Because theories can be incorrect, scientific generalization is not a perfect process. Formulating a theory is not a mathematical or statistical process, so generalization should not be considered a statistical exercise. It is really no more nor less than the process of causal inference itself.

It is curious that many people believe that generalizing from an epidemiologic study involves a mechanical process of making an inference about a target population of which the study population is considered a sample. This type of generalization does exist, in the field of survey sampling. In survey sampling, researchers draw samples from a larger population to avoid the expense of studying the entire population. In survey sampling, the statistical representativeness of the sample is the main concern for generalizing to the source population.

Nevertheless, while survey sampling is an important tool for characterizing a population efficiently, it does not always share the same goals as science. Survey sampling is useful for problems such as trying to predict how a population will vote in an election or what type of laundry soap the people in a region prefer. These are characteristics that depend on attitudes and for which there is little coherent biologic theory on which to base a scientific generalization. For this reason, survey results may be quickly outdated (election polls may be repeated weekly or even daily) and do not apply outside of the populations from which the surveys were conducted. (Disclaimer: I am not saying that social science is not science or that we cannot develop theories about social behavior. I am saying only that surveys about the current attitudes of a specific group of people are not the same as social theories.) Epidemiologic results, in contrast, seldom need to be repeated weekly to see if they still apply. A study conducted in Chicago that shows that exposure to ionizing radiation causes cancer does not need to be repeated in Houston to see if ionizing radiation also causes cancer in people living in Houston. Generalization about ionizing radiation and cancer is based on an understanding of the underlying biology rather than on statistical sampling.

It may be helpful to consider the problem of scientific generalization about causes of cancer from the viewpoint of a biologist studying carcinogenesis in mice. Most researchers study cancer, whether it be in mice, rats, rabbits, hamsters, or humans, because they would like to understand better the causes of human cancer. But if scientific generalization depended on having studied a statistically representative sample of the target population, researchers using mice would have nothing to contribute to the understanding of human cancer. They certainly do not study representative samples of people; they do not even study representative samples of mice. Instead, they seek mice that have uniformly similar genes and perhaps certain biologic characteristics. In choosing mice to study, they have to consider mundane issues such as the cost of the mice. Although researchers using animals are unlikely to worry about whether their mouse or hamster or rabbit subjects are statistically representative of all mice or hamsters or rabbits, they might consider whether the biology of the animal population they are studying is similar to (and in that sense representative of) that of humans. This type of representativeness, however, is not statistical representativeness based on sampling from a source population; it is a biologic representativeness based on scientific knowledge. Indeed, despite the absence of statistical representativeness, no one seriously doubts the contribution that animal research can make to the understanding of human disease.

Of course, many epidemiologic activities do require surveys to characterize a specific population, but these activities are usually examples of applied epidemiology as opposed to the science of epidemiology. In applied epidemiology, we use general epidemiologic knowledge and apply it to specific settings. In epidemiologic science, just as in laboratory science, we move away from the specific toward the general: we hope to generalize from research findings, a process based more on scientific knowledge, insight, and even conjecture about nature than on the statistical representativeness of the actual study participants. This principle has important implications for the design and interpretation of epidemiologic studies, as we shall see in Chapter 5.

Questions

1. Criticize the following statement: The cause of tuberculosis is infection with the tubercle bacillus.

2. A trait in chickens called yellow shank occurs when a specific genetic strain of chickens is fed yellow corn. Farmers who own only this strain of chickens observe the trait to depend entirely on the nature of the diet, that is, whether they feed their chickens yellow corn. Farmers who feed all of their chickens only yellow corn but own several strains of chicken observe the trait to be genetic. What argument could you use to explain to both kinds of farmer that the trait is both environmental and genetic?

3. A newspaper article proclaims that diabetes is neither genetic nor environmental but multicausal. Another article announces that half of all colon cancer cases are linked to genetic factors. Criticize both messages.

4. Suppose a new treatment for a fatal disease defers the average time of death among those with the disease for 20 years beyond the time that they would have otherwise died. Is it proper to say that this new treatment reduces the risk of death, or does it merely postpone death?

5. It is typically more difficult to study an exposure–disease relation that has a long induction period than one that has a short induction period. What difficulties ensue because the exposure–disease induction period is long?

6. Suppose that both A and B are causes of a disease that is always fatal so that the disease can only occur once in a single person. Among people exposed to both A and B, what is the maximum proportion of disease that could be attributed to either A or B alone? What is the maximum for the sum of the amount attributable to A and the amount attributable to B? Suppose that A and B exert their causal influence only in different causal mechanisms so that they never act in the same mechanism. Would that change your answer?

7. Adherents of induction claim that we all use this method of inference every day. We assume, for example, that the sun will rise tomorrow as it has in the past. Critics of induction claim that this knowledge is based on belief and assumption and is no more than a psychologic crutch. Why should it matter to a scientist whether scientific reasoning is based on induction or on a different approach, such as conjecture and refutation?

8. Give an example of competing hypotheses for which an epidemiologic study would provide a refutation of at least one.

9. Could a causal association fail to show evidence of a biologic gradient (Hill's fifth criterion)? Explain.

10. Suppose you are studying the influence of socioeconomic factors on cardiovascular disease. Would the study be more informative if (1) the study participants had the same distribution of socioeconomic factors as the general population or (2) the study participants were recruited so that there were equal numbers in each category of the socioeconomic variable(s)? Why?

References

1. Rothman, KJ: Causes. *Am J Epidemiol* 1976;104:587–592.
2. Higginson, J: Proportion of cancer due to occupation. *Prev Med* 1980; 9:180–188.
3. Ephron, E: *The Apocalyptics. Cancer and the Big Lie.* New York: Simon and Schuster, 1984.
4. Rothman, KJ: Induction and latent period. *Am J Epidemiol* 1981;114:253–259.
5. Mill, JS: *A System of Logic, Ratiocinative and Inductive,* 5th ed. London: Parker, Son and Bowin, 1862.
6. Magee, B: *Philosophy and the Real World. An Introduction to Karl Popper.* La Salle, IL: Open Court, 1985.
7. Hill, AB: The environment and disease: association or causation? *Proc R Soc Med* 1965;58:295–300.
8. US Department of Health, Education and Welfare. *Smoking and Health: Report of the Advisory Committee to the Surgeon General of the Public Health Service,* Public Health Service Publication 1103. Washington, D.C.: Government Printing Office, 1964.

3

Measuring Disease Occurrence and Causal Effects

As in most sciences, measurement is a central feature of epidemiology. Epidemiology has been defined as the study of the occurrence of illness.[1] The broad scope of epidemiology today demands a correspondingly broad interpretation of illness, to include injuries, birth defects, health outcomes, and other health-related events and conditions. The fundamental observations in epidemiology are measures of the occurrence of illness. In this chapter, we discuss several measures of disease frequency: *risk, incidence rate,* and *prevalence.* We also examine how these fundamental measures can be used to obtain derivative measures that aid in quantifying potentially causal relations between exposure and disease.

Measures of Disease Occurrence

Risk and Incidence Proportion

The concept of *risk* for disease is widely used and readily understood by many people. It is measured on the same scale and interpreted in the same way as a probability. In epidemiology, we often speak about risk applying to an individual, in which case we are describing the probability that a person will develop a given disease. It is usually pointless, however, to measure risk in a single person, since for most diseases we would say that the person either did or did not get the disease. Among a larger group of people, we could describe the proportion who developed the disease. If a population has N people and A people out of the N develop disease during a period of time, the proportion A/N represents the average risk of disease in the population during that period.

$$\text{Risk} = \frac{A}{N} = \frac{\text{Number of subjects developing disease during a time period}}{\text{Number of subjects followed for the time period}}$$

The measure of risk requires that all of the N people are followed for the entire time period during which the risk is being measured. The average risk in a group is also referred to as the *incidence proportion*. Often the word *risk* is used in reference to a single person and *incidence proportion* is used in reference to a group of people. Because we use averages taken from populations to estimate the risk experienced by individuals, we often use the two terms synonymously. We can use risk or incidence proportion to assess the onset of disease, death from a given disease, or any event that marks a health outcome.

One of the primary advantages of using risk as a measure of disease frequency is the extent to which it is readily understood by many people, including those who have little familiarity with epidemiology. To make risk useful as a technical or scientific measure, however, we need to clarify the concept. Suppose you read in the newspaper that women who are 60 years of age have a 2% risk of dying from cardiovascular disease. What does this statement mean? If you consider the possibilities, you may soon realize that the statement as written cannot be interpreted. It is certainly not true that a typical 60-year-old woman has a 2% chance of dying from cardiovascular disease within the next 24 hours or in the next week or month. A 2% risk would be high even for 1 year, unless the women in question have one or more characteristics that put them at unusually high risk compared with most 60-year-old women. The risk of developing fatal cardiovascular disease over the remaining lifetime of 60-year-old women, however, would likely be well above 2%. There might be some period of time over which the 2% figure would be correct, but any other period of time would imply a different value for the risk.

The only way to interpret a risk is to know the length of the time period over which the risk applies. This time period may be short or long, but without identifying it, risk values are not meaningful. Over a very short time period, the risk of any particular disease is usually extremely low. What is the probability that a given person will develop a given disease in the next 5 minutes? It is close to zero. The total risk over a period of time may climb from zero at the start of the period to a maximum theoretical limit of 100%, but it cannot decrease with time. Figure 3–1 illustrates two different possible patterns of risk during a 20-year interval. In pattern A, the risk climbs rapidly early during the period and then plateaus, whereas in pattern B, the risk climbs at a steadily increasing rate during the period.

How might these different risk patterns occur? As an example, a pattern similar to A might occur if a person who is susceptible to an infectious disease becomes immunized, in which case the leveling off of risk would not be gradual but sudden. Another way that a pattern like A might occur is if those who come into contact with a susceptible person become immunized, reducing the person's risk of acquiring the disease. A pattern similar to B might occur if a person has been exposed to a cause and is nearing the end of the typical induction time for the causal

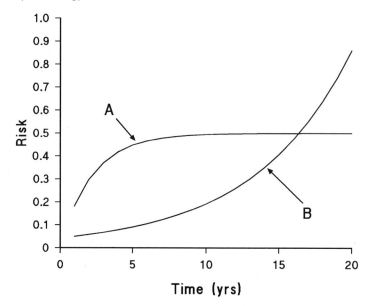

Figure 3–1. Two possible patterns of disease risk with time.

action, such as the risk of adenocarcinoma of the vagina among young women who were exposed to diethylstilbestrol while they were fetuses, discussed in Chapter 2. Another situation that can give rise to pattern B is simply the aging process, which often leads to sharply increasing risks as people progress beyond middle age.

Risk carries an important drawback as a tool for assessing the occurrence of illness: over any appreciable time interval, it is usually technically impossible to measure risk. The reason is a practical one: if a population is followed over a period of time, some people in the population will die from causes other than the outcome under study.

Suppose that you are interested in measuring the occurrence of domestic violence in a population of 10,000 married women over a 30-year period. Unfortunately, not all of the 10,000 women will survive the 30-year period. Some may die from extreme instances of domestic violence, but many more are likely to die from cardiovascular disease, cancer, infection, vehicular injury, and other causes. What if a woman died after 5 years of being followed without having been a victim of domestic violence? We could not say that she would not have been a victim of domestic violence during the subsequent 25 years. If we count her as part of the denominator, N, we will end up with an underestimate of the risk of domestic violence in a population of women who do survive 30 years. To see why, imagine that there are many women who do not survive the 30-year follow-up period. It is likely that among them there would be some who would have experienced domestic violence if they had instead survived. Thus, if we count these women who die during the follow-up period in the denominator, N, of a risk measure, then the numerator, A, which gives the number of cases of domestic violence, will be underestimated because A is supposed to represent the number of victims of domestic violence among a population of women followed for a full 30 years. In contrast, if we happen to be studying the risk of death from any cause, there would be no possibility of anyone dying from a cause that we were not measuring. Nevertheless, outside of studying death from any cause, it will always be possible for someone to die before the end of the follow-up period without experiencing the event that we are measuring.

This phenomenon of people being removed from a study through death from other causes is sometimes referred to as *competing risks*. Over a short period of time, the influence of competing risks is generally small, and it is not unusual for studies to ignore competing risks if the follow-up is short. For example, in the experiment in 1954 in which the Salk vaccine was tested, hundreds of thousands of schoolchildren were given either the Salk vaccine or a placebo. All of the children were followed for 1 year to assess the vaccine efficacy. Because only a small proportion of school-age children died from competing causes during the year of the study, it was reasonable to report the results of the Salk vaccine trial in terms of the observed risks. When study participants are older or are followed for longer periods of time, competing risks are greater and may need to be taken into account.

A related issue that affects long-term follow-up is *loss to follow-up*. Some people may be hard to track, to assess whether they have developed disease. They may move away or choose not to participate further in a research study. The difficulty in interpreting studies in which there have been losses to follow-up is sometimes similar to that of interpreting studies in which there are strong competing risks. In both situations, the researcher lacks complete follow-up of a study group for the intended period of follow-up.

Because of competing risks, it is often useful to think of risk or incidence proportion as hypothetical in the sense that it usually cannot be directly observed in a population. If competing risks did not occur and we could avoid all losses to follow-up, we could measure incidence proportion directly by dividing the number of observed cases by the number of people in the population followed. As mentioned above, if we study death from any cause as our outcome, there will be no competing risk; any death that occurs will count in the numerator of the risk measure. Most attempts to measure disease risk, however, are aimed at more specific outcomes or at disease onset rather than death. For such outcomes, there will always be competing risks. If one chooses to report the fraction A/N, which is the observed number of cases divided by the number of people who were initially being followed, it will underestimate the incidence proportion that would have been observed if there had been no competing risk.

Attack rate and case fatality rate

A term for risk or incidence proportion that is sometimes used in connection with infectious outbreaks is *attack rate*. An attack rate is simply the incidence proportion, or risk, of becoming afflicted with a condition during an epidemic period. For example, we might speak of an influenza epidemic with an attack rate of 10%, which means that 10% of the population developed the disease during the epidemic period. The time reference for an attack rate is usually not stated but implied by the biology of the disease being described. It is seldom measured in periods of more than a few months. A *secondary attack rate* is the attack rate among susceptible people who come into direct contact with *primary cases,* the cases infected in the initial wave of an epidemic.

Another version of the incidence proportion that is encountered frequently in clinical medicine is the *case fatality rate*. The case fatality rate is the proportion of people, among those who develop a disease, who then proceed to die from the disease. Thus, the population at risk when a case fatality rate is used is the population of people who have already developed the disease. The event being measured is not development of the disease but rather death from the disease (sometimes all deaths among patients, rather than just deaths from the disease, are counted). The case fatality rate is seldom accompanied by a specific time referent, which sometimes makes it difficult to interpret. It is typically used, and easiest to interpret, as a description of the proportion of people who succumb from an infectious disease, such as measles. The case fatality rate for measles in the United States is about 1.5 per 1000 cases. The time period for this risk of death is the comparatively short time frame in which measles infects an individual, ending in either recovery, death, or some other complication. For diseases that continue to affect a person over long periods of time, such as multiple sclerosis, it is more difficult to interpret a measure such as case fatality rate, and other types of mortality or survival measures are used instead.

Incidence Rate

To address the problem of competing risks, epidemiologists often resort to a different measure of disease occurrence, the *incidence rate*. This measure is similar to incidence proportion in that the numerator is the same. It is the number of cases, A, that occur in a population. The denominator, however, is different. Instead of dividing the number of cases by the number of people who were initially being followed, we divide the number of cases by a measure of time. This time measure is the summation, across all individuals, of the time experienced by the population being followed.

$$\text{Incidence rate} = \frac{A}{\text{Time}} = \frac{\text{Number of subjects developing disease}}{\text{Total time experienced for the subjects followed}}$$

One way to obtain this measure is to sum the time that each person is followed for every member of the group being followed. If a population is being followed for 30 years and a given person dies after 5 years of follow-up, then that person would contribute only 5 years to the sum for the group. Others might contribute more or fewer years, up to a maximum of the full 30 years of follow-up.

There are two methods of counting the time of an individual who develops the disease being measured. These methods depend on whether the disease or event can recur. Suppose that the disease is an upper respiratory tract infection, which can occur more than once in the same person. As a result, the numerator of an incidence rate could contain more than one occurrence of an upper respiratory tract infection from a single person. The denominator, then, should include all of the time that each person was at risk of getting any of these bouts of infection. In this situation, the time of follow-up for each person continues after that person recovers from an upper respiratory tract infection. On the other hand, if the event is death from leukemia, a person can be counted as a case only once. For someone who dies from leukemia, the time that would count in the denominator of an incidence rate would be the interval that begins at the start of follow-up and ends at death from leukemia. If a person can experience an event only once, the person ceases to contribute follow-up time after the event occurs.

In many situations, epidemiologists study events that could occur more than once in an individual but count only the first occurrence of the event. For example, researchers might count the occurrence of the first heart attack in an individual and ignore (or study separately) second or later heart attacks. Whenever only the first occurrence of a disease is of interest, the time contribution of a person to the denominator of an incidence rate will end when the disease occurs. The unifying concept in how to tally the time for the denominator of an incidence rate is simple: the time that goes into the denominator corresponds to the time experienced by the people being followed during which the disease or event being studied could have occurred. For this reason, the time tallied in the denominator of an incidence rate is often referred to as the *time at risk of disease*. The time in the denominator of an incidence rate should include every moment in which a person being followed is at risk for an event that would get tallied in the numerator of the rate. For events that cannot recur, once a person experiences the event, that person will have no more time at risk for disease, so the follow-up ends with the disease occurrence. The same is true of a person who dies from a competing risk.

The following diagram illustrates the time at risk for five hypothetical people being followed to measure the mortality rate of leukemia. (A *mortality rate* is an incidence rate in which the event being measured is death.) Only the first of the five people died from leukemia during the follow-up period. This person's time at risk ended with his or her death from leukemia. The second person died from another cause, an automobile crash, after which he or she was no longer at risk of dying from leukemia. The third person was lost to follow-up early during the follow-up period. Once a person is lost, if that person dies from leukemia, the death cannot be counted in the numerator of the rate because the researcher will not know about it. Therefore, the time at risk to be counted as a case in the numerator of the rate ends when a person becomes lost to follow-up. The last two people were followed for the complete period of follow-up. The total time that would be tallied in the denominator of the mortality rate for leukemia for these five people would correspond to the sum of the lengths of the five line segments in Figure 3–2.

Incidence rates treat one unit of time as equivalent to another, regardless of whether these time units come from the same person or from different people. The incidence rate measure is the ratio of cases to the total time at risk of disease. This ratio does not have the same simple interpretability as the risk measure. Let us compare the risk and incidence rate measures to see how they differ.

Whereas the incidence proportion, or risk, measure can be interpreted as a probability, the incidence rate cannot. First of all, unlike a proba-

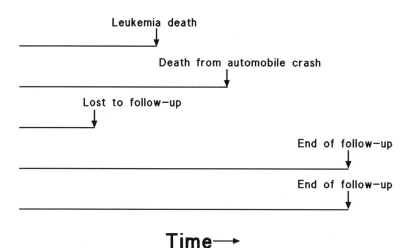

Time⟶

Figure 3–2. Time at risk for leukemia death for five people.

Table 3–1. Comparison of incidence proportion (risk) and incidence rate

Property	Incidence Proportion	Incidence Rate
Smallest value	0	0
Greatest value	1	Infinity
Units (dimensionality)	None	1/time
Interpretation	Probability	Inverse of waiting time

bility, the incidence rate does not even have the range of [0,1]. Instead, it can theoretically become as great as infinity. At first, it may seem puzzling that a measure of disease occurrence can exceed 1; after all, how can more than 100% of a population be affected? The answer is simply that the incidence rate does not measure the proportion of the population that is affected. It measures the ratio of the number of cases to the time at risk for disease. Because the denominator is measured in time units, we can always imagine that the denominator of an incidence rate could be smaller, making the rate larger. In fact, the numerical value of the incidence rate depends on what time unit is chosen. Suppose that we measure an incidence rate in a population as 47 cases occurring in 158 months. To make it clear that the time tallied in the denominator of an incidence rate is the sum of the time contribution from various people, we often refer to these time values as *person-time.* Accordingly, we might restate the preceding incidence rate as follows.

$$\frac{47 \text{ cases}}{158 \text{ person-months}} = \frac{0.30 \text{ cases}}{\text{person-month}}$$

We could restate this same incidence rate using person-years instead of person-months.

$$\frac{47 \text{ cases}}{13.17 \text{ person-years}} = \frac{3.57 \text{ cases}}{\text{person-year}}$$

The above two expressions measure the same incidence rate; the only difference is the time unit chosen to express the denominator. The different time units affect the numerical values. The situation is much the same as expressing speed in different units of time or distance. For example, 60 miles/hour is the same as 88 feet/second or 26.84 meters/second. The change in units results in a change in the numerical value. The analogy between incidence rate and speed is helpful in understanding other aspects of incidence rate. One important concept is that incidence rate, like speed, is an instantaneous concept. Imagine driving along a highway. At any instant, you and your vehicle have a certain speed. The speed can change from moment to moment. The speedometer gives you a continuous measure of the current speed. Suppose that the speed is expressed in terms of kilometers/hour. Although the time unit for the denominator is 1 hour, it does not require an hour to measure the speed of the vehicle. You can note the speed for a given instant from the speedometer (which continuously calculates the ratio of distance to time over a recent finite short interval of time). Similarly, an incidence rate is the momentary rate at which cases are occurring within a group of people. To measure an incidence rate takes a finite amount of time, just as it does to measure speed; but the concepts of speed and incidence rate can be thought of as applying at a given instant. Thus, if an incidence rate is measured, as is often the case, with person-years in the denominator, the rate nevertheless might apply to an instant rather than to a year. Similarly, speed expressed in kilometers/hour does not necessarily apply to an hour but perhaps to an instant. The point is that for both measures, the unit of time in the denominator is arbitrary and has no implication for any period of time over which the rate is measured or applies.

One commonly finds incidence rates expressed in the form of 50 cases per 100,000 and described as "annual incidence." This is a clumsy description of an incidence rate, equivalent to describing an instantaneous speed in terms of an "hourly distance." Nevertheless, we can translate this phrasing to correspond with what we have already described for incidence rates. We could express this rate as 50 cases per 100,000 person-years or, equivalently, $50/100,000 \text{ yr}^{-1}$. (The negative 1 in the exponent means inverse, implying that the denominator of the fraction is measured in units of years.)

Whereas the risk measure has a clear interpretation for epidemiologists and non-epidemiologists alike (provided that a time period for the risk is specified), incidence rate does not appear to have a clear interpretation. It is difficult to conceptualize a measure of occurrence that takes the ratio of events to the total time in which the events occur. Nevertheless, under certain conditions, there is an interpretation that we can give to an incidence rate. The dimensionality of an incidence rate is that of the reciprocal of time, which is just another way of saying that in an incidence rate the only units involved are time units, which appear in the denominator. Suppose we invert the incidence rate. Its reciprocal is measured in units of time. To what time does the reciprocal of an incidence rate correspond? Under steady-state conditions, a situation in which rates do not change with time, the reciprocal of the incidence rate equals the average time until an event occurs. This time is referred to as the *waiting time*. Take as an example the incidence rate above of 3.57 cases per person-year. Let us write this rate as 3.57 yr^{-1}. (The cases in the numerator of an incidence rate do not have any units.) If we take the reciprocal of this rate, we obtain $1/3.57$ years $= 0.28$ years. This value can be interpreted as an average waiting time of 0.28 years until the occurrence of the first event that the rate measures. As another example, consider a mortality rate of 11 deaths per 1000 person-years, which we could also write as $11/1000 \text{ yr}^{-1}$. If this is the total mortality rate for an entire population, then the waiting time that corresponds to it would represent the average time until death. The average time until death is also referred to as the "expectation of life," or expected survival time. If we take the reciprocal of $11/1000 \text{ yr}^{-1}$, we obtain 90.9 years, which would be interpretable as the expectation of life for a population in a steady state that had a mortality rate of $11/1000 \text{ yr}^{-1}$. Unfortunately, mortality rates typically change with time over the time scales that apply to this example. Consequently, taking the reciprocal of the mortality rate for a population is not a practical method for estimating the expectation of life. Nevertheless, it is helpful to understand what kind of interpretation we might assign to an incidence rate or a mortality rate, even if the conditions that justify the interpretation are often not applicable.

Chicken and egg

An old riddle asks "If a chicken and one-half lays an egg and one-half in a day and one-half, then how many eggs does one chicken lay in one day?" This riddle is a rate problem. The question amounts to asking "What is the rate of egg-laying expressed in eggs per chicken-day?" To get the answer, we express the rate as the number of eggs in the numerator and the number of chicken-days in the denominator, so we have 1.5 eggs/(1.5 chickens·1.5 days) = 1.5 eggs/2.25 chicken-days. This calculation gives a rate of ⅔ egg per chicken-day, so the answer to the riddle is ⅔.

Relation Between Risk and Incidence Rate

Because the interpretation of risk is so much more straightforward than that of incidence rate, it is often convenient to convert incidence rate measures into risk measures. Fortunately, this conversion is usually not difficult. The simplest formula to convert an incidence rate to a risk is as follows.

$$\text{Risk} = \text{Incidence rate} \times \text{Time} \qquad (3\text{--}1)$$

It is a good habit when applying an equation such as 3–1 to check the dimensionality of each expression and make certain that both sides of the equation are equivalent. In this case, risk is measured as a proportion and has no dimensions. Although risk applies for a specific period of time, the time period is a descriptor for the risk but not part of the measure itself. Risk has no units of time or any other quantity built in, but is interpreted as a probability. The right side of equation 3–1 is the product of two quantities, one of which is measured in units of the reciprocal of time and the other of which is simply time itself. This product has no dimensionality either, so the equation holds as far as dimensionality is concerned.

In addition to checking the dimensionality, it is useful to check the range of the measures in an equation such as 3–1. Note that risk is a pure number in the range [0,1]. Values outside this range are not permitted. In contrast, incidence rate has a range of [0,∞], and time has a range of [0,∞] as well. Therefore, the product of incidence rate and time will not have a range that is the same as risk; the product can easily exceed 1. This analysis tells us that equation 3–1 is not applicable throughout the entire range of values for incidence rate and time. In more general terms, equation 3–1 is an approximation that works well as long as the risk calculated on the left is less than about 20%. Above that value, the approximation worsens.

Let us consider an example of how this equation works. Suppose that we have a population of 10,000 people who experience an incidence rate of lung cancer of 8 cases per 10,000 person-years. If we followed the population for 1 year, equation 3–1 tells us that the risk of lung cancer would be 8 in 10,000 for the 1-year period (the product of 8/10,000 person-years and 1 year), or 0.0008. If the same rate were experienced for only half a year, then the risk would be half of 0.0008, or 0.0004. Equation 3–1 calculates risk as directly proportional to both the incidence rate and the time period, so as the time period is extended, the risk becomes proportionately greater.

Now suppose that we have a population of 1000 people who experience a mortality rate of 11 deaths per 1000 person-years for a 20-year period. Equation 3–1 predicts that the risk of death over 20 years would be $11/1000 \text{ yr}^{-1} \times 20 \text{ yr} = 0.22$, or 22%. In other words, equation 3–1 predicts that among the 1000 people at the start of the follow-up, there will be 220 deaths during the 20 years. The 220 deaths are the sum of 11 deaths that occur among 1000 people every year for 20 years. This calculation neglects the fact that the size of the population at risk of death shrinks gradually as deaths occur. If we took the shrinkage into account, we would not end up with 220 deaths at the end of 20 years, but fewer.

Table 3–2 describes how many deaths would be expected to occur during each year of the 20 years of follow-up if the mortality rate of $11/1000 \text{ yr}^{-1}$ were applied to a population of 1000 people for 20 years. The table shows that at the end of 20 years we would actually expect about 197 deaths rather than 220 because a steadily smaller population is at risk of death each year. The table also shows that the prediction of 11 deaths per year from equation 3–1 is a good estimate for the early part of the follow-up, but that gradually the number of deaths expected becomes considerably lower than the estimate. Why is the number of expected deaths not quite 11 even for the first year, in which there are

Table 3–2. Number of expected deaths over 20 years among 1000 people experiencing a mortality rate of 11 deaths per 1000 person-years

Year	Expected Number Alive at Start of Year	Expected Deaths	Cumulative Deaths
1	1000.000	10.940	10.940
2	989.060	10.820	21.760
3	978.240	10.702	32.461
4	967.539	10.585	43.046
5	956.954	10.469	53.515
6	946.485	10.354	63.869
7	936.131	10.241	74.110
8	925.890	10.129	84.239
9	915.761	10.018	94.257
10	905.743	9.909	104.166
11	895.834	9.800	113.966
12	886.034	9.693	123.659
13	876.341	9.587	133.246
14	866.754	9.482	142.728
15	857.272	9.378	152.106
16	847.894	9.276	161.382
17	838.618	9.174	170.556
18	829.444	9.074	179.630
19	820.370	8.975	188.605
20	811.395	8.876	197.481

1000 people being followed at the start of the year? As soon as the first death occurs, the number of people being followed is less than 1000, and the number of expected deaths is consequently influenced. As seen in Table 3–2, the expected deaths decline gradually throughout the period of follow-up.

If we extended the calculations in the table further, the discrepancy between the risk calculated from equation 3–1 and the expected risk would grow. Figure 3–3 graphs the cumulative total of deaths that would be expected and the number projected from equation 3–1 over 50 years of follow-up. Initially, the two curves are close, but as the cumulative risk of death rises, they diverge. The bottom curve in the figure is an exponential curve, related to the curve that describes *exponential decay:* if a population experiences a constant rate of death, the proportion remaining alive follows an exponential curve with time. This exponential decay is the same curve that describes radioactive decay. If a population of radioactive atoms converts from one atomic state to another at a constant rate, the proportion of atoms left in the initial state follows the curve of exponential decay. Strictly speaking, the lower curve in Figure 3–3 is the complement of an exponential decay curve. Instead of show-

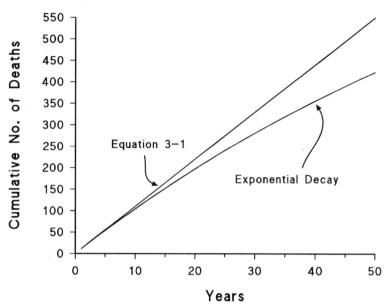

Figure 3–3. Cumulative number of deaths in 1000 people experiencing a mortality rate of 11 deaths per 1000 person-years, presuming no population shrinkage (*equation 3–1*) and taking the population shrinkage into account (*exponential decay*).

ing the decreasing number remaining alive (which would be the curve of exponential decay), it shows the increasing number who have died, which is the total number in the population minus the number remaining alive. Given enough time, this curve gradually flattens out so that the total number of deaths approaches the total number of people in the population. The curve based on equation 3–1, in contrast, continues to predict 11 more deaths each year regardless of how many people remain alive, and eventually it would predict a cumulative number of deaths that exceeds the original size of the population.

Clearly, we cannot use equation 3–1 to calculate risks that are large because it is a poor approximation in such situations. For many epidemiologic applications, however, the calculated risks are reasonably small and equation 3–1 is perfectly adequate for calculating risks from incidence rates.

Equation 3–1 calculates risk for a time period over which a single incidence rate applies. The calculation assumes that the incidence rate, an instantaneous concept, remains constant over the time period. What if the incidence rate changes with time, as would often be the case? In that event, one can still calculate risk, but separately for subintervals of the time period. Each of the time intervals should be short enough so that the incidence rate applied to it can be considered approximately constant. The shorter the intervals, the better the overall accuracy of the risk calculation. On the other hand, it is impractical to use many short intervals unless there are adequate data to obtain meaningful incidence rates for each interval.

The method of calculating risks over a time period with changing incidence rates is known as *survival analysis*. It can be applied to nonfatal risks as well as to death but the approach originated from data that related to deaths. To implement the method, one creates a table similar to Table 3–2, called a *life-table*. The purpose of a life-table is to calculate the probability of surviving through each successive time interval that constitutes the period of interest. The overall survival probability is equal to the cumulative product of the probabilities of surviving through each successive interval, and the overall risk is equal to 1 minus the overall probability of survival.

Table 3–3 is a simplified life-table that enables us to calculate the risk of dying from a motor-vehicle injury,[2] based on applying the mortality rates to a hypothetical group of 100,000 people followed from birth through age 85. In this example, the time periods correspond to age intervals. As is often true of life-table calculations, it is assumed that there is no competing risk from other causes. The number initially at risk has been arbitrarily set at 100,000 people. Mortality rates are then used to calculate how many deaths occur among those remaining at risk in each age interval. This calculation is strictly hypothetical because the number at risk is reduced only by deaths from motor-vehicle injury. All other causes of death are ignored. The risk for each age interval can be calculated by applying the mortality rate to the time interval. The number of deaths and the number remaining at risk are not needed for this calculation but are included to show how the initial group would shrink slightly as some people are lost to fatal motor-vehicle accidents. The complement for the risk in each age category is the survival probability, calculated as 1 minus the risk. The cumulative product of the survival probabilities for each successive age category is the overall probability of surviving from birth through that age interval without dying from a

Table 3–3. Life-table for death from motor-vehicle injury from birth through age 85 (mortality rates are deaths per 100,000 person-years)

Age (years)	Mortality Rate	At Risk	Deaths in Interval	Risk	Survival Probability	Cumulative Survival Probability
0–14	4.7	100,000	70.5	0.000705	0.999295	0.999295
15–24	35.9	99,930	358.1	0.003584	0.996416	0.995714
25–44	20.1	99,571	399.5	0.004012	0.995988	0.991719
45–64	18.4	99,172	364.3	0.003673	0.996327	0.988077
65–84	21.7	98,808	427.9	0.004331	0.995669	0.983798

Adapted from Iskrant and Joliet, table 24[2]

motor-vehicle accident. Because all other causes of death have been ignored, this survival probability is conditional on the absence of competing risks. If we subtract the final cumulative survival probability from 1, we obtain the total risk, from birth until the 85th birthday, of dying from a motor-vehicle accident. This risk is $1 - 0.9838 = 1.6\%$. It assumes that everyone will live to the 85th birthday if not for the occurrence of motor-vehicle accidents, so it overstates the actual proportion of people who will die in a motor-vehicle accident before they reach age 85. Another assumption is that these mortality rates, which have been gathered from a cross-section of the population at a given time, would apply to a group of people over the course of 85 years of life. If the mortality rates changed with time, the risk estimated from the life-table would be inaccurate.

Because the overall risk of motor-vehicle death calculated from the rates in Table 3–3 is low, a simpler approach would have worked nearly as well. The simpler method applies equation 3–1 repeatedly to each age group, without subtracting the deaths from the total population at risk.

Risk from birth until age 85 of dying from a motor-vehicle injury =

$$\frac{4.7}{100,000 \text{ yr}} (15 \text{ yr}) + \frac{35.9}{100,000 \text{ yr}} (10 \text{ yr}) + \frac{20.1}{100,000 \text{ yr}} (20 \text{ yr})$$

$$+ \frac{18.4}{100,000 \text{ yr}} (20 \text{ yr}) + \frac{21.7}{100,000 \text{ yr}} (20 \text{ yr})$$

$$= \frac{4.7(15) + 35.9(10) + 20.1(20) + 18.4(20) + 21.7(20)}{100,000} = 1.6\%$$

This result is same as the one obtained using a life-table approach. This method is often used to estimate lifetime risks for many diseases, such as suicide, cancer, or heart disease.

Point-Source and Propagated Epidemics

An *epidemic* is an unusually high occurrence of disease. The definition of "unusually high" may differ depending on the circumstances, so there is no clear demarcation between an epidemic and a smaller fluctuation. Furthermore, the high occurrence could represent an increase in the occurrence of a disease that still occurs in the population in the absence of an epidemic, although less frequently than during the epidemic, or it may represent an *outbreak*, which is a sudden increase in the occurrence of a disease that is usually absent or nearly absent (Fig. 3–4).

If an epidemic stems from a single source of exposure to a causal agent, it is considered a *point-source epidemic*. Examples of point-source epidemics would be food poisoning of restaurant patrons who had been served contaminated food, or cancer among survivors of the atomic

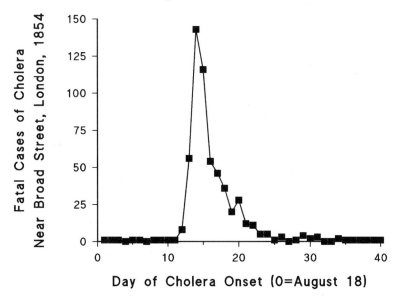

Figure 3–4. Epidemic curve of fatal cholera cases during the Broad Street outbreak, London 1854.[3]

bomb blasts in Hiroshima and Nagasaki. Although the time scales of these epidemics differ dramatically along with the nature of the diseases and their causes, both have in common that all people would have been exposed to the same causal component that produced the epidemic, either the contaminated food in the restaurant or the ionizing radiation from the bomb blast. The exposure in a point-source epidemic is typically newly introduced into the environment, thus accounting for the epidemic.

Typically, the shape of the epidemic curve of a point-source epidemic shows an initial steep increase in the incidence rate followed by a more gradual decline (often described as log-normal). The asymmetry of the curve stems partly from the fact that biologic curves with a meaningful zero point tend to be asymmetrical because there is less variability in the direction of the zero point than in the other direction. (If the zero point is sufficiently far from the modal value, the asymmetry may not be apparent, as in the distribution of birth weights.) For example, the distribution of recovery times for a wound to heal will be log-normal. Similarly, the distribution of induction times until the occurrence of illness after a common exposure will be log-normal.

An example of an asymmetrical epidemic curve is that of the 1854 cholera epidemic described by John Snow.[3] In that outbreak, exposure to contaminated water in the neighborhood of the water pump at Broad Street in London produced a log-normal epidemic curve (Fig. 3–4). Snow is renowned for having convinced local authorities to remove the handle from the pump, but they did so only on September 8, when the epidemic was well past its peak and the number of cases was already declining.

Another factor that may affect the shape of an epidemic curve is the way in which the curve is calculated. It is common, as in Figure 3–4, to plot the number of new cases instead of the incidence rate among susceptible people. People who have already succumbed to an infectious disease may no longer be susceptible to it for some period of time. If a substantial proportion of a population is affected by the outbreak, the number of susceptible people will decline gradually as the epidemic progresses and the attack rate increases. This change in the susceptible population will lead to a more rapid decline over time in the number of new cases than in the incidence rate. The incidence rate will decline more slowly than the number of new cases because in the incidence rate the declining number of new cases is divided by a dwindling amount of susceptible person-time.

A *propagated epidemic* is one in which the causal agent is itself transmitted through a population. Influenza epidemics are propagated by person-to-person transmission of the virus. The epidemic of lung cancer during the twentieth century was a propagated epidemic attributable to the spread of tobacco smoking through many cultures and societies. The curve for a propagated epidemic tends to show a more gradual initial rise and a more symmetrical shape than that for a point-source epidemic because the causes spread gradually through the population.

Although we may think of point-source epidemics as occurring over a short time span, they do not always occur over shorter time spans than propagated epidemics. The epidemic of cancer attributable to exposure to the atomic bombs in Hiroshima and Nagasaki was a point-source epidemic that began a few years after the explosions and continues into the present. Another possible point-source epidemic that occurred over decades was an apparent outbreak of multiple sclerosis in the Faroe Islands, which followed the occupation of those islands by British troops during the Second World War.[4] Furthermore, propagated epidemics can occur over extremely short time spans. One example is epidemic hysteria, a disease often propagated from person to person in minutes. An example of an epidemic curve for a hysteria outbreak is depicted in Figure 3–5. In this epidemic, 210 elementary school children developed symptoms of headache, abdominal pain, and nausea. These symptoms were attributed by the investigators to hysteric anxiety.[5]

Prevalence Proportion

Both incidence proportion and incidence rate are measures that assess the frequency of disease onset. The numerator of either measure is the frequency of events that are defined as the occurrence of disease. In contrast, *prevalence proportion*, often simply referred to as *prevalence*, does not measure disease onset. Instead, it is a measure of disease status.

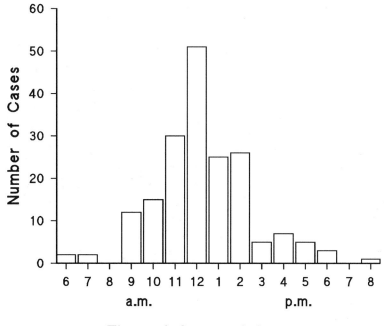

Time of Onset of Symptoms

Figure 3–5. Epidemic curve of an outbreak of hysteria in elementary school children, November 6, 1985.

The simplest way of considering disease status is to consider disease either present or absent. The prevalence proportion is the proportion of people in a population that has disease. Consider a population of size N, and suppose that P individuals in the population have disease at a given time. The prevalence proportion will be P/N. For example, suppose that among 10,000 female residents of a town on July 1, 2001, 1200 have hypertension. The prevalence proportion of hypertension among women in the town on that date is $1200/10,000 = 0.12$, or 12%. This prevalence applies only to the point in time July 1, 2001. Prevalence can change with time as the factors that affect prevalence change.

What factors affect prevalence? Clearly, disease occurrence affects prevalence. The greater the incidence of disease, the more people will have it. But prevalence is also related to the length of time that a person has disease. The longer the duration of disease once it occurs, the higher the prevalence. Diseases with short duration may have a low prevalence even if the incidence rate is high. One reason is that if the disease is benign, there may be a rapid recovery. Thus, the prevalence of upper respiratory infection may be low despite a high incidence because after a brief period most people recover from the infection and are no longer in the disease state. Duration may also be short for a grave disease that leads to rapid death. Thus, the prevalence of aortic hemorrhage would be low even if it had a high incidence, because it generally leads to death within minutes. What the low prevalence means is that at any given moment, there will be only an extremely small proportion of people who are at that moment suffering from an aortic hemorrhage. Some diseases have a short duration because either recovery or death ensues promptly; appendicitis is an example. Other diseases have a long duration because one cannot recover from them, but they are compatible with a long survival (although the survival is often shorter than it would be without the disease). Diabetes, Crohn's disease, multiple sclerosis, parkinsonism, and glaucoma are examples.

Because prevalence reflects both incidence rate and disease duration, it is not as useful as incidence for studying the causes of disease. It is extremely useful, however, for measuring the disease burden on a population, especially if those who have the disease require specific medical attention. For example, the prevalent number of people in a population with end-stage renal disease predicts the need in that population for dialysis facilities.

In a *steady state*, which is a situation in which incidence rates and disease duration are stable over time, the prevalence proportion, P, will have the following relation to the incidence rate.

$$\frac{P}{1 - P} = I\bar{D} \tag{3-2}$$

In equation 3–2, I is the incidence rate and $\bar{D}$ is the average duration of disease. The quantity $P/(1 - P)$ is known as the *prevalence odds*. In general, whenever we take a proportion, such as prevalence proportion, and divide it by 1 minus the proportion, the resulting ratio is referred to as the *odds* for that proportion. If a horse is a 3-to-1 favorite at a race track, it means that the horse is thought to have a probability of winning of 0.75. The odds of the horse winning is $0.75/(1 - 0.75) = 3$, usually described as 3 to 1. Similarly, if a prevalence proportion is 0.75, the prevalence odds would be 3, and a prevalence of 0.20 would correspond to a prevalence odds of $0.20/(1 - 0.20) = 0.25$. For small prevalences, the value of the prevalence proportion and the prevalence odds will be close because the denominator of the odds expression will be close to 1. Therefore, for small prevalences, say less than 0.1, we could rewrite equation 3–2 as follows.

$$P \doteq I\bar{D} \tag{3-3}$$

Equation 3–3 indicates that, given a steady state and a low prevalence, prevalence is approximately equal to the product of the incidence rate and the mean duration of disease.

As we did earlier for risk and incidence rate, it is useful to check the equation to make certain that the dimensionality and ranges of both sides are satisfied. For dimensionality, we find that the right-hand side of equations 3–2 and 3–3 involves the product of a time measure, disease duration, with incidence rate, which has units that are the reciprocal of time. The product is dimensionless, a pure number. Prevalence proportion, like risk or incidence proportion, is also dimensionless, which satisfies the dimensionality requirements for both equations 3–2 and 3–3. The range of incidence rates and mean durations of illness, however, is $[0,\infty]$, because there is no upper limit to either. Equation 3–3 does not satisfy the range requirement because the prevalence proportion on the left side of the equation, like any proportion, has a range of $[0,1]$. That is the reason that equation 3–3 is applicable only to small values of prevalence. The prevalence odds in equation 3–2, however, has a range of $[0,\infty]$, and is applicable for all values rather than just for small values of the prevalence proportion. We can rewrite equation 3–2 to solve for the prevalence proportion as follows.

$$P = \frac{I\bar{D}}{1 + I\bar{D}} \tag{3-4}$$

As mentioned above, prevalence is used to measure the disease burden in a population. This type of epidemiologic application relates more to administrative areas of public health than to causal research. Nevertheless, there are research areas in which prevalence measures are used more commonly than incidence measures. One of these is the area of birth defects. When we describe the occurrence of congenital malformations among live-born infants in terms of the proportion of these infants who have a malformation, we use a prevalence measure. For example, the proportion of infants who are born alive with a defect of the ventricular septum of the heart is a prevalence. It measures the status of live-born infants with respect to the presence or absence of a ventricular septal defect. To measure the incidence rate or incidence proportion of ventricular septal defects would require the ascertainment of a population of embryos who were at risk to develop the defect, and measurement of the defect's occurrence among these embryos. Such data are usually not obtainable because many pregnancies end before the pregnancy is detected, so the population of embryos is not readily identified. Even when a woman knows she is pregnant, if the pregnancy ends early, information about the pregnancy may never come to the attention of researchers. For these reasons, incidence measures for birth defects are uncommon. Prevalence at birth is easier to assess and often used as a substitute for incidence measures. Although easier to obtain, prevalence measures have a drawback when used for causal research: factors that increase prevalence may do so not by increasing the occurrence of the condition but by increasing the duration of the condition. Thus, a factor associated with the prevalence of ventricular septal defect at birth could be a cause of ventricular septal defect, but it could also be a factor that does not cause the defect but instead enables embryos that develop the defect to survive until birth.

Prevalence is also sometimes used in research to measure diseases that have insidious onset, such as diabetes or multiple sclerosis. These are conditions for which it may be difficult to define onset, and it therefore may be necessary in some settings to describe the condition in terms of prevalence rather than incidence.

Prevalence of characteristics

Because prevalence measures status, it is often used to describe the status of characteristics or conditions other than disease in a population. For example, the proportion of a population that engages in cigarette smoking would often be described as the prevalence of smoking. The proportion of a population exposed to a given agent is often referred to as the exposure prevalence. Prevalence could be used to describe the proportion of people in a population with brown eyes, type O blood, or an active driver's license. Because epidemiology relates many individual and population characteristics to disease occurrence, it often employs prevalence measures to describe the frequency of these characteristics.

Measures of Causal Effects

A central objective of epidemiologic research is to study the causes of disease. How should we measure the effect of exposure to determine whether exposure causes disease? In a courtroom, experts are asked to opine whether the disease of a given patient has been caused by a specific exposure. This approach of assigning causation in a single person is radically different from the epidemiologic approach, which does not attempt to attribute causation in any individual instance. Rather, the epidemiologic approach is to evaluate the proposition that the exposure is a cause of the disease in a theoretical sense, rather than in a specific person.

An elementary but essential principle that epidemiologists must keep in mind is that a person may be exposed to an agent and then develop disease without there being any causal connection between exposure and disease. For this reason, we cannot consider the incidence proportion or the incidence rate among exposed people to measure a causal effect. Indeed, there might be no effect or even a preventive effect of exposure. For example, if a vaccine does not confer perfect immunity, then some vaccinated people will get the disease that the vaccine is intended to prevent. The occurrence of disease among vaccinated people is not a sign that the vaccine is causing the disease, because the disease will occur even more frequently among unvaccinated people. It is merely a sign that the vaccine is not a perfect preventive. To measure a causal effect, we have to contrast the experience of exposed people with what would have happened in the absence of exposure.

The Counterfactual Ideal

It is useful to consider how we might measure causal effects in an ideal way. People differ from one another in myriad ways. If we compare risks or incidence rates between exposed and unexposed people, we cannot be certain that the differences in risk or rate are attributable to the exposure. Instead, they could be attributable to other factors that differ between exposed and unexposed people. We may be able to measure and take into account some of these other factors, but others may elude us, hindering any definite inference. Even if we matched people who were exposed with similar people who were not exposed, they might still differ in unapparent ways. The ideal comparison would be of people with themselves in both an exposed and an unexposed state. Such a comparison envisions the impossible goal of matching each person with himself or herself, being exposed in one incarnation and unexposed in the other. If such an impossible goal were achievable, it would allow us to know the effect of exposure, because the only difference between the two settings would be the exposure. Because this situation is not realistic, it is called *counterfactual.*

The counterfactual goal posits not only a comparison of a person with himself or herself but also a repetition of the experience during the same time. That is, some studies actually do pair the experiences of a person under both exposed and unexposed conditions. The experimental version of such studies is called a *crossover study* because the study subject crosses over from one study group to the other after a period of time. Although crossover studies come close to the ideal of a counterfactual comparison, they do not achieve it because a person can be in only one study group at a given time. The time sequence may affect the interpretation, and the passage of time means that the two experiences may differ by factors other than the exposure. Thus, the counterfactual setting is truly impossible, as it implies that a person relives the same experience twice, once with exposure and once without.

In the theoretical ideal of a counterfactual study, each exposed person would be compared with his or her unexposed counterfactual experience. The incidence proportion among exposed people could be compared with the incidence proportion among the counterfactual unexposed. Any difference in these proportions would have to be an effect of exposure. Suppose we observed 100 exposed people and found that in 1 year 25 developed disease, for an incidence proportion of 0.25. We would theoretically like to compare this experience with the counterfactual, unobservable experience of the same 100 people going through the same year under the same conditions, except for their being unexposed. Suppose that in those conditions 10 developed disease. Then the incidence proportion for comparison would be 0.10. The difference, 15 cases in 100 during the year, or 0.15, would be a measure of the causal effect of the exposure.

Effect Measures

Because we can never achieve the counterfactual ideal, we strive to come as close as possible in the design of epidemiologic studies. Instead of comparing the experience of an exposed group with its counterfactual ideal, we must compare that experience with that of a real unexposed population. The goal is to find an unexposed population that would give a result close, if not identical, to that from a counterfactual comparison.

Suppose we consider the same 100 exposed people mentioned above, among whom 25 get the disease in 1 year. As a substitute for their missing counterfactual experience, we seek the experience of 100 unexposed persons who can provide an estimate of what would have occurred among the exposed had they not been exposed. This substitution is the crucial concern in many epidemiologic studies: does the experience of the unexposed group actually simulate what would have happened to the exposed group had they been unexposed? If we observe 10 cases of disease in the unexposed group, how can we know that the difference between the 25 cases in the exposed group and the 10 in the unexposed group is attributable to the exposure? Perhaps the exposure has no effect, but the unexposed group is at a lower risk for disease than the exposed group. What if we had observed 25 cases in both the exposed and the unexposed groups? The exposure might have no effect, but it might also have a strong effect that is balanced by the fact that the unexposed group has a higher risk for disease.

To achieve a valid substitution for the counterfactual experience, we resort to various design methods that promote comparability. The crossover study is one example, which promotes comparability by comparing the experience of each exposed person to himself or herself at a different time. This approach will be feasible only if the exposure can be studied in an experimental setting and if it has a brief effect. Another approach is a randomized experiment. In these studies, all participants are randomly assigned to the exposure groups. Given enough randomized participants, we can expect the distributions of other characteristics in the exposed and unexposed groups to be similar. Other approaches might involve choosing unexposed study subjects who have the same or similar risk-factor profiles for disease as the exposed subjects. However the comparability is achieved, its success is the overriding concern for any epidemiologic study that aims at evaluating a causal effect.

If we can assume that the exposed and unexposed groups are otherwise comparable with regard to risk for disease, we can compare measures of disease occurrence to assess the effect of the exposure. The two most commonly compared measures are the incidence proportion, or risk, and the incidence rate. The *risk difference* would be the difference in incidence proportion or risk between the exposed and unexposed groups. If the incidence proportion is 0.25 for the exposed and 0.10 for the unexposed, then the risk difference would be 0.15. With an incidence rate instead of a risk to measure disease occurrence, we can likewise calculate the *incidence rate difference* for the two measures.

Difference measures such as risk difference and incidence rate difference measure the absolute effect of an exposure. It is also possible to measure the relative effect. As an analogy, consider how one might assess the performance of an investment over a period of time. Suppose that an initial investment of $100 became $120 after 1 year. One might take the difference in the value of the investment at the end of the year and at the beginning as a measure of how well the investment did. This difference, $20, measures the absolute performance of the investment. The relative performance is obtained by dividing the absolute increase by the initial amount, which gives $20/$100, or 20%. Contrast this investment experience with that of another investment, in which an initial sum of $1000 grew to $1150 after 1 year. For the latter investment, the absolute increment is $150, far greater than the $20 from the first investment. On the other hand, the relative performance of the second investment is $150/$1000, or 15%, which is worse than the first investment.

We can obtain relative measures of effect in the same manner that we figure the relative success of an investment. We first obtain an absolute measure of effect, which would be either the risk difference or the incidence rate difference, and then we divide that by the measure of occurrence of disease among the unexposed. For risks, the relative effect is

$$\text{Relative effect} = \frac{\text{Risk difference}}{\text{Risk in unexposed}} = \frac{RD}{R_0}$$

[RD is the risk difference, and R_0 is the risk among the unexposed. Because $RD = R_1 - R_0$ (R_1 is the risk among exposed), this expression can be rewritten as follows.

$$\text{Relative effect} = \frac{RD}{R_0} = \frac{R_1 - R_0}{R_0} = RR - 1 \qquad (3\text{--}5)$$

where the *risk ratio (RR)* is defined as R_1/R_0. Thus, the relative effect is the risk ratio minus 1. This result is exactly parallel to the investment analogy, in which the relative success of the investment was the ratio of the value after investing divided by the value before investing, minus 1.

For the smaller of the two investments, this computation would give ($120/$100) − 1 = 1.2 − 1 = 20%. If we have a risk in exposed of 0.25 and a risk in unexposed of 0.10, then the relative effect is (0.25/0.10) − 1, or 1.5 (sometimes expressed as 150%). The RR is 2.5, and the relative effect is the part of the RR in excess of 1.0. The value of 1.0 is the value of RR when there is no effect. By defining the relative effect in this way, we ensure that we have a relative effect of 0 when the absolute effect is also 0.

Because the relative effect is simply $RR − 1$, it is common for epidemiologists to refer to the RR itself as a measure of relative effect, without subtracting the 1. When the RR is used in this way, it is important to keep in mind that a value of 1 corresponds to the absence of an effect. For example, RR of 3 represents twice as great an effect as RR of 2. Sometimes epidemiologists refer to the percentage increase in risk to convey the magnitude of relative effect. For example, one might describe an effect that represents a 120% increase in risk. Obviously, this increase is meant to describe a relative, not an absolute, effect because we cannot have an absolute effect of 120%. Describing an effect in terms of a percentage increase in risk is precisely the same as the relative effect defined above. An increase of 120% corresponds to RR of 2.2, which is 2.2 − 1.0 = 120% greater than 1. Thus, the 120% is a description of the relative effect that subtracts the 1 from the RR. Usually, it is straightforward to determine from the context whether a description of relative effect is RR or $RR − 1$. If the effect is described as a fivefold increase in risk, it means that the RR is 5. If the effect is described as a 10% increase in risk, it will correspond to RR of 1.1, which is 1.1 − 1.0.

Effect measures that involve the incidence rate difference and the incidence rate ratio are defined analogously to those involving the risk difference and the risk ratio. Table 3–4 compares absolute and relative measures constructed from risks and rates.

The range of the risk difference measure derives from the range of risk itself, which is [0,1]. The lowest possible risk difference would result from an exposed group with zero risk and an unexposed group at 100% risk, giving −1 for the difference. Analogously, the greatest possible risk difference, 1, comes from an exposed group with 100% risk and an unexposed group with zero risk. Risk difference has no dimensionality (that is, it has no units and is measured as a pure number) because the underlying measure, risk, is also dimensionless and the dimensionality of a difference is the same as that of the underlying measure.

The risk ratio has a range that is never negative because a risk cannot be negative. The smallest risk ratio occurs when the risk in the exposed group, the numerator of the risk ratio, is zero. The largest risk ratio occurs when the risk among the unexposed is zero, giving a ratio of infinity. Any ratio measure will be dimensionless if the numerator and denominator quantities have the same dimensionality because the di-

Table 3–4. Comparison of absolute and relative effect measures

Measure	Numerical Range	Dimensionality
Risk difference	$[-1, +1]$	None
Risk ratio	$[0, \infty]$	None
Incidence rate difference	$[-\infty, +\infty]$	1/time
Incidence rate ratio	$[0, \infty]$	None

mensions divide out. In the case of risk ratio, both the numerator and the denominator, as well as their ratio, are dimensionless.

Incidence rates range from zero to infinity and have the dimensionality of 1/time. From these characteristics, it is straightforward to deduce the range and dimensionality of the incidence rate difference and the incidence rate ratio.

Examples

Table 3–5 presents data on the risk of diarrhea among breast-fed infants during a 10-day period following their infection with *Vibrio cholerae 01,* according to the level of antipolysaccharide antibody titers in their mother's breast milk.[6] The data show a substantial difference in the risk of developing diarrhea according to whether the mother's breast milk contains a low or a high level of antipolysaccharide antibody. The risk difference for infants exposed to milk with low compared with high levels of antibody is $0.86 - 0.44 = 0.42$. This risk difference reflects the additional risk of diarrhea among infants whose mother's breast milk has low antibody titers compared with the risk among infants whose mother's milk has high titers, under the assumption that the infants exposed to low titers would experience a risk equal to that of those exposed to high titers except for the lower antibody levels.

Table 3–5. Diarrhea during a 10-day follow-up period in breast-fed infants colonized with *Vibrio cholera 01* by the level of antipolysaccharide antibody titer in their mother's breast milk*

	Antibody Level		
	Low	High	Total
Diarrhea	12	7	19
No diarrhea	2	9	11
Total	14	16	30
Risk	0.86	0.44	0.63

*Data from Glass et al.[6]

We can also measure the effect of breast-feeding on diarrhea risk in relative terms. The *RR* is 0.86/0.44 = 1.96. The relative effect is 1.96 − 1, or 0.96, which would be expressed as a 96% greater risk of diarrhea among infants exposed to low antibody titers in the mother's breast milk. Commonly, we would simply describe the risk among infants exposed to low titers as being 1.96 times the risk among infants exposed to high titers.

The calculation of effects from incidence rate data is analogous to the calculation of effects from risk data. Table 3–6 gives data for the incidence rate of breast cancer among women who were treated for tuberculosis early in the twentieth century.[7] Some women received a treatment that involved repeated fluoroscopy of the lungs, with a resulting high dose of ionizing radiation to the chest.

The incidence rate among those exposed to radiation is $14.6/10,000 \ \text{yr}^{-1}$ compared with $7.9/10,000 \ \text{yr}^{-1}$ among those unexposed. The incidence rate difference is $(14.6 - 7.9)/10,000 \ \text{yr}^{-1} = 6.7/10,000 \ \text{yr}^{-1}$. This difference reflects the rate of breast cancer among exposed women that can be attributed to radiation exposure, under the assumption that exposed women would have had a rate equal to that among unexposed women if not for the exposure. As before, we can also measure the effect in relative terms. The incidence rate ratio is 14.6/7.9, or 1.86. The relative effect is 1.86 − 1, or 0.86, which would be expressed as an 86% greater rate of breast cancer among women exposed to the radiation. Alternatively, one might simply describe the incidence rate ratio as indicating a rate of breast cancer among exposed women that is 1.86 times that of the rate among unexposed women.

Relation Between Risk Ratios and Rate Ratios

Risk data produce estimates of effect that are either risk differences or risk ratios, and rate data produce estimates of effect that are rate differences or rate ratios. Risks cannot be compared directly with rates (they have different units), and for the same reason risk differences cannot be

Table 3–6. Breast cancer cases and person-years of observation for women with tuberculosis repeatedly exposed to multiple x-ray fluoroscopies and unexposed women with tuberculosis*

| | *Radiation Exposure* | | |
	Yes	**No**	**Total**
Breast cancer cases	41	15	56
Person-years	28,010	19,017	47,027
Rate (cases/10,000 person-yr)	14.6	7.9	11.9

*Data from Boice and Monson.[7]

Rounding: How many digits should be reported?

A frequent question that arises in the reporting of results is how many digits of accuracy should be reported. In some published papers, a risk ratio might be reported as 4.1; in others, the same number might be reported as 4.0846. It is clear that the number of digits should reflect the amount of precision in the data. The number 4.0846 implies that one is fairly sure that the data warrant a reported value that lies between 4.084 and 4.085. Only a truly large study would produce that level of precision. Nevertheless, it is surprisingly hard to offer a general rule for the number of digits that should be reported. For example, suppose one believes that for a given study reporting should carry into the first decimal, say, 4.1. If the study reported risk ratios, however, and these took on values below 1.0, the ratios would be rounded to values such as 0.7 or 0.8. This amount of rounding error is greater, in proportion to the size of the effect, than the rounding error in a reported value such as 4.1. So a simple rule such as one decimal place (or two, or whatever) will not suffice. How about the rule that suggests using a constant number of meaningful digits? With this rule, 4.1 would have the same reporting accuracy as 0.83. This rule may appear to be an improvement, but it breaks down near the value of 1.0 for ratio measures: it suggests that we should distinguish 0.98 from 0.99, but that we should not distinguish 1.00 from 1.01. Both of the latter numbers would be rounded to 1.0, and the next reportable value would be 1.1. If all of the risk ratios to be reported ranged from 0.9 to 1.1, this rule would make little sense.

No rule is needed as long as the writer uses good judgment and thinks about the number of digits to report. One should remember never to round values used in intermediate calculations; round only in the final step before reporting. Also, consider that rounding 1.41 to 1.4 is not a large error, but rounding 1.25 to 1.2 or to 1.3 is a rounding error that amounts to 20% of the effect for a rate ratio (keeping in mind that 1.0 equals no effect). Finally, when rounding a number ending in 5, it is customary to round upward, but it is preferable to use an unbiased strategy, such as rounding to the nearest even number. Thus, under this strategy, both 1.75 and 1.85 would be rounded to 1.8.

---

compared with rate differences. Under certain conditions, however, a risk ratio will be equivalent to a rate ratio. Suppose that we have incidence rates that are constant over time, with the rate among exposed people equal to I_1 and the rate among unexposed people equal to I_0. From equation 3–1, we know that a constant incidence rate will result in a risk approximately equal to the product of the rate times the time period, provided that the time period is short enough so that the risk remains under about 0.20. Above that value, the approximation does not work very well. Suppose that we are dealing with short time periods. Then the ratio of the risk among the exposed to the risk among the unexposed, R_1/R_0, will be expressed as follows.

$$\text{Risk ratio} = \frac{R_1}{R_0} = \frac{I_1 \cdot \text{Time}}{I_0 \cdot \text{Time}} = \frac{I_1}{I_0}$$

This relation shows that the risk ratio will be the same as the rate ratio, provided that the time period over which the risks apply is sufficiently short or the rates are sufficiently low for equation 3–1 to apply. The shorter the time period or the lower the rates, the better the approximation represented by equation 3–1 and the closer the value of the risk ratio to the rate ratio. Over longer time periods (the length depending on the value of the rates involved), risks may become sufficiently great that the risk ratio will begin to diverge from the rate ratio. Because risks cannot exceed 1.0, the maximum value of a risk ratio cannot be greater than 1 divided by the risk among the unexposed. Consider the data in Table 3–5, for example. The risk in the high antibody group (which we consider to be the unexposed group) is 0.44. With this risk for the unexposed group, the risk ratio cannot exceed 1/0.44, or 2.3. In fact, the observed risk ratio of 1.96 is not far below the maximum possible risk ratio. Incidence rate ratios are not constrained by this type of ceiling, so when the unexposed risk is high, we can expect there to be a divergence between the incidence rate ratio and the risk ratio. We do not know the incidence rates that gave rise to the risks illustrated in Table 3–5, but it is reasonable to infer that the ratio of the incidence rates, were they available, would be much greater than 1.96.

If the time period over which a risk is calculated approaches 0, the risk itself also approaches 0: thus, the risk of a given person having a myocardial infarction may be 10% in a decade, but in the next 10 seconds it will be extremely small, its value shrinking along with the length of the time interval. Nevertheless, the ratio of two quantities that both approach 0 does not necessarily approach 0; in the case of the risk ratio calculated for risks that apply to shorter and shorter time intervals, as the risks approach 0, the risk ratio approaches the value of the incidence rate ratio. The incidence rate ratio is thus the limiting value for the risk ratio as the time interval over which the risks are taken approaches 0. Therefore, we can describe the incidence rate ratio as an *instantaneous risk ratio*. This equivalence of the two types of ratio for short time intervals has resulted in some confusion of terminology: often, the phrase *relative risk* is used to refer to either an incidence rate ratio or a risk ratio. Either of the latter terms is preferable to *relative risk*, since they describe the nature of the data from which the ratio derives. Nevertheless, because the risk ratio and the rate ratio are equivalent for small risks, the more general term *relative risk* has some justification. Thus, the often-used notation *RR* is sometimes read to mean relative risk, which might equally be read as risk ratio or rate ratio, all of which are equivalent if the risks are sufficiently small.

When risk does not mean risk

In referring to effects, some speakers or writers inaccurately use the word *risk* in place of the word *effect*. For example, suppose that a study reports two risk ratios for lung cancer from asbestos exposure, 5.0 for young adults and 2.5 for older adults. One might occasionally see these effect values described as follows: "The risk of lung cancer from asbestos exposure is not as great among older people as among younger people." This statement is incorrect. In fact, the risk difference between those exposed and those unexposed to asbestos is sure to be greater among older adults than younger adults, and thus the risk attributable to the effect of asbestos is greater in older adults. The risk ratio is smaller among older adults because the risk of lung cancer increases steeply with age, so the ratio for older adults is based on a larger denominator. The statement is wrong because the term *risk* has been used in place of the term *risk ratio*, or the more general term *effect*. It is perfectly correct to describe the data as follows: "The risk ratio of lung cancer from asbestos exposure is not as great among older people as among younger people."

Attributable Fraction

If we take the risk difference between exposed and unexposed people, $R_1 - R_0$, and divide it by the risk in the unexposed group, we obtain the relative measure of effect (see equation 3–5 above). We can also divide the risk difference by the risk in exposed people to get an expression that we refer to as the attributable fraction.

$$\text{Attributable fraction} = \frac{RD}{R_1} = \frac{R_1 - R_0}{R_1} = 1 - \frac{1}{RR} = \frac{RR - 1}{RR} \qquad (3\text{–}6)$$

If the risk difference reflects a causal effect that is not distorted by any bias, then the attributable fraction is a measure that quantifies the proportion of the disease burden among exposed people that is caused by the exposure. To illustrate, consider the hypothetical data in Table 3–7. The risk of disease during a 1-year period is 0.05 among the exposed and 0.01 among the unexposed. Let us suppose that this difference can be reasonably attributed to the effect of the exposure (because we believe that we have accounted for all substantial biases). The risk difference is 0.04, which is 80% of the risk among the exposed. We would then say that the exposure accounts for 80% of the disease that occurs among

Table 3–7. Hypothetical data giving 1-year disease risks for exposed and unexposed people

	Unexposed	Exposed	Total
Disease	900	500	1400
No disease	89,100	9500	98,600
Total	90,000	10,000	100,000
Risk	0.01	0.05	0.014

exposed people during the 1-year period. Another way to calculate the attributable fraction is from the risk ratio: $(5 - 1)/5 = 80\%$.

If we wish to calculate the attributable fraction for the entire population of 100,000 people in Table 3–7, we would first calculate the attributable fraction for exposed people. To obtain the overall attributable fraction for the total population, the fraction among the exposed should be multiplied by the proportion of all cases in the total population that is exposed. There are 1400 cases in the entire population, of whom 500 are exposed. Thus, the proportion of exposed cases is $500/1400 = 0.357$. The overall attributable fraction for the population is the product of the attributable fraction among the exposed and the proportion of exposed cases: $0.8 \times 0.357 = 0.286$. That is, 28.6% of all cases in the population are attributable to the exposure. This calculation is based on a straightforward idea: no case can be caused by exposure unless the person is exposed, so among all of the cases, only some of the exposed cases can be attributable to the exposure. There were 500 exposed cases, of whom we calculated that 400 represent excess cases caused by the exposure. None of the 900 cases among the unexposed is attributable to the exposure, so among the total of 1400 cases in the population, only 400 of the exposed cases are attributable to the exposure: the proportion $400/1400 = 0.286$, which is the same value that we calculated.

If the exposure is categorized into more than two levels, we can use formula 3–7, which takes into account each of the exposure levels.

$$\text{Total attributable fraction} = \sum_i (AF_i \times P_i) \qquad (3\text{–}7)$$

AF_i is the attributable fraction for exposure level i, P_i represents the proportion of all cases that falls in exposure category i, and Σ indicates the sum of each of the exposure-specific attributable fractions. For the unexposed group, the attributable fraction would be 0.

Let us apply formula 3–7 to the hypothetical data in Table 3–8, which give risks for a population with three levels of exposure. The attributable fraction for the group with no exposure is 0. For the low-exposure group, the attributable fraction is 0.50 because the risk ratio is 2. For the

Table 3–8. Hypothetical data giving 1-year disease risks for people at three
levels of exposure

	Exposure			
	None	**Low**	**High**	**Total**
Disease	100	1200	1200	2500
No disease	9900	58,800	28,800	97,500
Total	10,000	60,000	30,000	100,000
Risk	0.01	0.02	0.04	0.025
Risk ratio	1.00	2.00	4.00	
Proportion of all cases	0.04	0.48	0.48	

high-exposure group, the attributable fraction is 0.75 because the risk
ratio is 4. The total attributable fraction is as follows.

$$0 + 0.50(0.48) + 0.75(0.48) = 0.24 + 0.36 = 0.60$$

The same result can also be calculated directly from the number of attributable cases at each exposure level.

$$(0 + 600 + 900)/2500 = 0.60$$

Under certain assumptions, the estimation of attributable fractions
can be based on rates as well as risks. Thus, in formula 3–6, which uses
the risk ratio to calculate the attributable fraction, the rate ratio could be
used instead, provided that the conditions are met for the rate ratio to
approximate the risk ratio. If exposure results in an increase in disease
occurrence at some levels of exposure and a decrease at other levels of
exposure, compared with no exposure, the net attributable fraction will
be a combination of the prevented cases and the caused cases at the
different levels of exposure. The net effect of exposure in such situations
can be difficult to assess and may obscure the components of the exposure effect. This topic is discussed in greater detail by Rothman and
Greenland.[8]

Questions

1. Suppose that in a population of 100 people 30 die. The risk of death
   could be calculated as 30/100. What is missing from this measure?
2. Can we calculate a rate for the data in question 1? If so, what is it? If
   not, why not?
3. Eventually all people die. Why should we not state that the mortality
   rate for any population is always 100%?
4. If incidence rates remain constant with time and if exposure causes
   disease, which will be greater, the risk ratio or the rate ratio?

5. Why is it incorrect to describe a rate ratio of 10 as indicating a high risk for disease among the exposed?
6. A newspaper article states that a disease has increased by 1200% in the past decade. What is the rate ratio that corresponds to this level of increase?
7. Another disease has increased by 20%. What is the rate ratio that corresponds to this increase?
8. From the data in Table 3–5, calculate the fraction of diarrhea cases among infants exposed to a low antibody level that is attributable to the low antibody level. Calculate the fraction of all diarrhea cases attributable to exposure to low antibody levels. What assumptions are needed to interpret the result as an attributable fraction?
9. What proportion of the 56 breast cancer cases in Table 3–6 is attributable to radiation exposure? What are the assumptions?
10. Suppose you worked for a health agency and had collected data on the incidence of lower back pain among people in different occupations. What measures of effect would you choose and why?
11. Suppose that the rate ratio measuring the relation between an exposure and a disease is 3 in two different countries. Would this situation imply that exposed people have the same risk in the two countries? Would it imply that the effect of the exposure is the same in the two countries? Why or why not?

References

1. Cole, P: The evolving case-control study. *J Chron Dis* 1979;32:15–27.
2. Iskrant AP, Joliet PV: Table 24 in *Accidents and Homicides* Vital and Health Statistics Monographs, American Public Health Association, Harvard University Press, Cambridge, 1968.
3. Snow, J: *On the Mode of Communication of Cholera*, 2nd ed. London: John Churchill, 1860. (Facsimile of 1936 reprinted edition by Hafner, New York, 1965.)
4. Kurtzke, JF, Hyllested, K: Multiple sclerosis in the Faroe Islands: clinical and epidemiologic features. *Ann Neurol* 1979;5:6–21.
5. Cole, TB, Chorba, TL, Horan, JM: Patterns of transmission of epidemic hysteria in a school. *Epidemiology* 1990;1:212–218.
6. Glass, RI, Svennerholm, AM, Stoll, BJ, et al: Protection against cholera in breast-fed children by antibiotics in breast milk. *N Engl J Med* 1983;308:1389–1392.
7. Boice, JD, Monson, RR: Breast cancer in women after repeated fluoroscopic examinations of the chest. *J Natl Cancer Inst* 1977;59:823–832.
8. Rothman, KJ, Greenland, S: *Modern Epidemiology*, 2nd ed. Philadelphia: Lippincott-Raven, 1998.

4

Types of Epidemiologic Study

In the last chapter, we learned about measures of disease frequency, including risk, incidence rate, and prevalence; measures of effect, including risk and incidence rate differences and ratios; as well as attributable fractions. Epidemiologic studies may be viewed as measurement exercises undertaken to obtain estimates of these epidemiologic measures. The simplest studies aim only at estimating a single risk, incidence rate, or prevalence. More complicated studies aim at comparing measures of disease occurrence, with the goal of predicting such occurrence, learning about the causes of disease, or evaluating the impact of disease on a population. This chapter describes the two main types of epidemiologic study, the cohort study and the case-control study, along with several variants.

Cohort Studies

In epidemiology, a *cohort* is defined most broadly as "any designated group of individuals who are followed or traced over a period of time." [1] A cohort study, which is the archetype for all epidemiologic studies, involves measuring the occurrence of disease within one or more cohorts. Typically, a cohort comprises persons with a common characteristic, such as an exposure or ethnic identity. For simplicity, we refer to two cohorts, *exposed* and *unexposed,* in our discussion. In this context, we use the term *exposed* in its most general sense; for example, an exposed cohort could have in common the presence of a specific gene. The purpose of following a cohort is to measure the occurrence of one or more specific diseases during the period of follow-up, usually with the aim of comparing the disease rates for two or more cohorts.

The concept of following a cohort to measure disease occurrence may appear straightforward, but there are many complications involving who is eligible to be followed, what should count as an instance of disease, how the incidence rates or risks are measured, and how exposure ought to be defined. Before we explore these issues, let us examine, as an example, an elegantly designed epidemiologic cohort study.

John Snow's Natural Experiment

In the last chapter, we looked at data compiled by John Snow regarding the cholera outbreak in London in 1854 (Fig. 3–4). In London at that time, there were several water companies that piped drinking water to residents. Snow's so-called "natural experiment" consisted of comparing the cholera mortality rates for residents subscribing to two of the major water companies, the Southwark and Vauxhall Company, which piped impure Thames water contaminated with sewage, and the Lambeth Company, which in 1852 changed its collection from opposite Hungerford Market upstream to Thames Ditton, thus obtaining a supply of water free of the sewage of London. Snow[2] described it, as follows.

> . . . the intermixing of the water supply of the Southwark and Vauxhall Company with that of the Lambeth Company, over an extensive part of London, admitted of the subject being sifted in such a way as to yield the most incontrovertible proof on one side or the other. In the subdistricts . . . supplied by both companies, the mixing of the supply is of the most intimate kind. The pipes of each company go down all the streets, and into nearly all the courts and alleys. A few houses are supplied by one company and a few by the other, according to the decision of the owner or occupier at the time when the Water Companies were in active competition. In many cases a single house has a supply different from that on either side. Each company supplies both rich and poor, both large houses and small; there is no difference in either the condition or occupation of the persons receiving the water of the different companies . . . it is obvious that no experiment could have been devised which would more thoroughly test the effect of water supply on the progress of cholera than this.
>
> The experiment, too, was on the grandest scale. No fewer than three hundred thousand people of both sexes, of every age and occupation, and of every rank and station, from gentle folks down to the very poor, were divided into two groups without their choice, and, in most cases, without their knowledge; one group being supplied with water containing the sewage of London, and amongst it, whatever might have come from the cholera patients, the other group having water quite free from impurity.
> To turn this experiment to account, all that was required was to learn the supply of water to each individual house where a fatal attack of cholera might occur. . . .

From this natural experiment, Snow was able to estimate the frequency of cholera deaths, using households as the denominator, separately for people in each of the two cohorts.

According to a return which was made to Parliament, the Southwark and Vauxhall Company supplied 40,046 houses from January 1 to December 31, 1853, and the Lambeth Company supplied 26,107 houses during the same period; consequently, as 286 fatal attacks of cholera took place, in the first four weeks of the epidemic, in houses supplied by the former company, and only 14 in houses supplied by the latter, the proportion of fatal attacks to each 10,000 houses was as follows: Southwark and Vauxhall 71, Lambeth 5. The cholera was therefore fourteen times as fatal at this period, amongst persons having the impure water of the Southwark and Vauxhall Company, as amongst those having the purer water from Thames Ditton.

Snow also obtained estimates of the size of the population served by the two water companies, enabling him to report the attack rate of fatal cholera among residents of households served by them during the 1854 outbreak (Table 4–1). Residents whose water came from the Southwark and Vauxhall Company had an attack rate 5.8 times greater than that of residents whose water came from the Lambeth Company.

Snow saw that circumstance had created conditions that emulated an experiment, in which people who were otherwise alike in relevant regards differed by their consumption of pure or impure water. In an actual experiment, the investigator assigns the study participants to the exposed and unexposed groups. In a natural experiment, as studies such as Snow's have come to be known, the investigator takes advantage of a setting that serves effectively as an experiment. One might argue that the role of the investigator in a natural experiment requires more creativity and insight than in an actual experiment. In the natural experiment, the investigator has to see the opportunity for the research and define the study populations to capitalize on the setting. For example, Snow conducted his study within specific neighborhoods in London where the pipes from these two water companies were intermingled. In other districts, there was less intermingling of pipes from the various water companies that supplied water to dwellings. Comparing the attack rates across various districts of London would have been a less

Table 4–1. Attack rate of fatal cholera among customers of the Southwark and Vauxhall Company (exposed cohort) and the Lambeth Company (unexposed cohort), London, 1854*

	Water Company	
	Southwark and Vauxhall	**Lambeth**
Cholera deaths	4,093	461
Population	266,516	173,748
Attack rate	0.0154	0.0027

*Data from Snow.[2]

persuasive way to evaluate the effect of the water supply because many factors differed from one district to another. Within the area in which the pipes of the Southwark and Vauxhall Company and those of the Lambeth Company were intermingled, however, Snow saw that there was little difference between those who consumed water from one company or the other, apart from the water supply itself. Part of his genius was identifying the precise setting in which to conduct the study.

Experiments

Experiments are conceptually straightforward. Experiments are cohort studies, although not all cohort studies are experiments. In epidemiology, an experiment is a study in which the incidence rate or the risk of disease in two or more cohorts is compared, after assigning the exposure to the people who comprise the cohorts. Moreover, in an experiment, the reason for the exposure assignment is solely to suit the objectives of the study; if people receive their exposure assignment based on considerations other than the study protocol, it is not a true experiment. (The *protocol* is the set of rules by which the study is conducted.)

Epidemiologic experiments are most frequently conducted in a clinical setting, with the aim of evaluating which treatment for a disease is better. Such studies are known as *clinical trials* (the word *trial* is used as a synonym for an epidemiologic experiment). All study subjects have been diagnosed with a specific disease, but that disease is not the disease event that is being studied. Rather, it is some consequence of that disease, such as death or spread of a cancer, that becomes the "disease" event studied in a clinical trial. The aim of a clinical trial is to evaluate the incidence rate of disease complications in the cohorts assigned to the different treatment groups. In most trials, treatments are assigned by *randomization,* using random number assignment. Randomization tends

---

Natural experiments are not experiments

In John Snow's natural experiment, customers of the Southwark and Vauxhall and the Lambeth Companies were not randomly assigned to their water supply. In fact, they were not assigned at all, as they would be in an experiment. The "natural experiment" is not an actual experiment but, rather, a cohort study that simulates what would occur in an experiment. In Snow's description of the customers of the two water companies, he gives the impression that the comparability between them was nearly as good as might have been achieved by random assignment. Thus, we have an experiment created by 'nature,' or a natural experiment, which might be more accurately described as a cohort study designed by an ingenious epidemiologist.

Table 4–2. Randomized trial comparing the risk of opportunistic infection among patients with a recent Human Immunodeficiency Virus infection who received either zidovudine or placebo

	Treatment Group	
	Zidovudine	Placebo
Opportunistic infection	1	7
Total patients	39	38
Risk	0.026	0.184

*Data from Kinloch-de Loes et al.[3]

to produce comparability between the cohorts with respect to factors that might affect the rate of complications.

The data in Table 4–2 come from a clinical trial of adult patients recently infected with human immunodeficiency virus, to determine whether early treatment with zidovudine was effective at improving the prognosis.[3] Patients were randomly assigned to receive either zidovudine or placebo and then followed for an average of 15 months. The data show that the risk of getting an opportunistic infection during the follow-up period was low among those who received early zidovudine treatment but considerably higher among those who received a dummy (placebo) treatment.

Not all epidemiologic experiments are clinical trials; they are merely the most common type of experiment. Epidemiologists also conduct *field trials,* which differ from clinical trials mainly in that the study participants are not patients. In a field trial, the goal is not to study the complications of an existing disease, but to study the primary prevention of a disease. For example, experiments of new vaccines to prevent infectious illness are field trials because the study participants have not yet been diagnosed with a particular disease. In a clinical trial, the study participants can be followed through regular clinic visits, whereas in a field trial it may be necessary to contact participants for follow-up directly at home, work, or school. The largest formal human experiment ever conducted, the Salk vaccine trial of 1954, is a prominent example of a field trial.[4] It was conducted to evaluate the efficacy of a new vaccine to prevent paralytic poliomyelitis and paved the way for the first widespread use of vaccination to prevent poliomyelitis.

Another type of experiment is a *community intervention trial.* In this type of study, the exposure is assigned to groups of people rather than singly. For example, the community fluoridation trials in the 1940s and 1950s that evaluated the effect of fluoride in a community water supply were community intervention trials. The data in Table 4–3 illustrate a community intervention trial that evaluated a program of home-based neonatal care and management of sepsis designed to prevent death

Table 4–3. Neonatal mortality in the third of 3 years after instituting a community intervention trial of home-based neonatal care in rural Indian villages*

	Intervention Group	
	Home Care	Usual Care
Infant deaths	38	64
Number of births	979	940
Risk	0.039	0.068

*Data from Bang et al.[5]

among infants in rural India.[5] This trial, as is often the case for community intervention trials, did not employ random assignment. Instead, the investigators selected 39 villages targeted for the new program and 47 villages in which the new program was not introduced. The program consisted of frequent home visits after each birth in the village by health workers who were trained for the study to deal with problems in neonatal care. This program resulted in reduced neonatal mortality for each of the 3 years of its implementation, with the reductions increasing with time. The data in Table 4–3 show the results for the third of the 3 years.

Population at Risk

Snow's study on cholera defined two cohorts on the basis of their water supply, one being the customers of the Southwark and Vauxhall Company, which drew polluted water from the lower Thames river, and the other being the customers of the Lambeth Company, which drew water from the comparatively pure upper Thames. Any person in either of these cohorts could have contracted cholera. Snow measured the rate of cholera occurrence among the people in each cohort.

To understand clearly which people can belong to a cohort in an epidemiologic study, we must consider a basic requirement for cohort membership: cohort members must meet the criteria for being at risk of disease. Indeed, the members of a cohort to be followed are sometimes described as the *population at risk.* The term implies that all members of the cohort should be at risk for developing the specific disease(s) being measured. As a consequence, determining who may be part of the population at risk may depend on which disease is being measured.

A standard requirement of any population at risk is that everyone be free of the disease being measured at the outset of follow-up. The reason is that one usually cannot develop anew a disease that one currently has. Thus, someone with diabetes cannot develop diabetes, and someone with schizophrenia cannot develop schizophrenia. To be at risk of disease implies that everyone in the population at risk must be alive at the start of follow-up; dead people are not at risk of getting any disease.

Being alive and free of the disease are straightforward eligibility conditions, but other eligibility conditions may not be as simple. Suppose that the outcome is the development of measles. Should people who have received a measles vaccination be included in the population at risk? If they are completely immunized, they are not at risk for measles. But how can one know if the vaccine has conferred complete immunity? In a cohort being studied for the occurrence of breast cancer, should men be considered part of the population at risk? Men do develop breast cancer, but it is rare compared with the occurrence in women. One solution is to distinguish male and female breast cancer as different diseases. In that case, if female breast cancer is being studied, males would be excluded from the population at risk.

Some diseases occur only once in a person, whereas others can recur. Death is the clearest example of a disease outcome that can occur but once to a given person. Other examples would include diabetes, multiple sclerosis, chickenpox, and cleft palate. Disease can occur only once if it is incurable or if recovery confers complete lifetime immunity. If the disease can occur only once, anyone in a cohort who develops the disease is no longer at risk of developing it again and, therefore, exits from the population at risk as soon as the disease occurs. Also, any person who dies during the follow-up period, for whatever reason, would no longer be part of a population at risk. The members of the population at risk at any given time must be people in whom the disease can still occur. It might be possible, however, for someone with a disease to recover from the disease and then to develop it again. For example, someone with a urinary tract infection can recover and then succumb to another urinary tract infection. In that case, the person would not be part of the population at risk while he or she has the urinary tract infection but could become part of the population at risk again at the time of recovery. Thus, being part of a population at risk is a dynamic process. People may enter and leave a population at risk depending on their health and other possible eligibility criteria (such as age or geography).

Cohort Study of Vitamin A During Pregnancy—An Example

To study the relation between diet and other exposures of pregnant women and the development of birth defects in their offspring, Milunsky and colleagues[6] interviewed more than 22,000 pregnant women early in their pregnancies. The original purpose was to study the potential preventive effect of folate in the diet in relation to a class of birth defects known as neural-tube defects. A later study, based on the same population of women, evaluated the role of dietary vitamin A in causing another class of birth defects that affected either the heart or the head, cranial neural-crest defects.[7] For the latter study, the women were divided into cohorts according to the amount of vitamin A in their diet, from food or supplements. The data in Table 4–4 summarize the results

---

Disease-free does not imply healthy

Although a population at risk should be free of disease at the outset of follow-up, it is incorrect to conclude that the population at risk is healthy. The requirement to be free of disease does not imply health; it merely implies that the people being followed do not have the specific disease(s) being measured. Indeed, the search for a population that is healthy in the sense of being free of all disease is fruitless. If *disease* is defined broadly, virtually every person has some disease at any given time: acne, periodontal disease, back ailments, allergies, vision deficits, obesity, asthma, and respiratory infection are examples of the prevalent conditions that make it nearly impossible to find even one person who may be said to be completely healthy. Being free of disease and therefore a member of a population at risk implies only that the person is free of the specific disease(s) being followed, not all diseases.

---

of this cohort study. The table shows that the prevalence of these defects increased steadily and substantially with increasing intake of vitamin A supplements by pregnant women.

Table 4–4 gives results for four separate cohorts of the study population, each defined according to the level of supplemental intake of vitamin A that the women reported in the interview. The occurrence of cranial neural-crest defects increased substantially for women who took supplements of vitamin A in doses greater than 8000 IU/day.

Closed and Open Cohorts

There are two types of cohort that epidemiologists follow. A *closed cohort* is one with a fixed membership. Once it is defined and follow-up begins, no one can be added to a closed cohort. The initial roster may dwindle, however, as people in the cohort die, are lost to follow-up, or develop the disease. Randomized experiments are examples of studies of closed cohorts; the follow-up begins at randomization, a starting point for ev-

Table 4–4. Prevalence of birth defects among the offspring of four cohorts of pregnant women, classified according to their intake of supplemental vitamin A during early pregnancy*

	Level of Vitamin A Intake from Supplements (IU/day)			
	0–5000	**5001–8000**	**8001–10,000**	**≥10,001**
Affected infants	51	54	9	7
Pregnancies	11,083	10,585	763	317
Prevalence	0.46%	0.51%	1.18%	2.21%

*Data from Rothman et al.[7]

eryone in the study. Another example of a closed cohort study is the landmark Framingham Heart Study, initiated in 1949 and continuing to the present.[8]

In contrast, an *open cohort*, which is also referred to as a *dynamic cohort* or a *dynamic population*, can take on new members as time passes. An example of an open cohort would be the population of Connecticut, which has one of the oldest cancer registries in the United States. The population studied in the Connecticut cancer registry may be considered a dynamic cohort that comprises the people of Connecticut. Cancer incidence rates over a period of time in Connecticut reflect the rate of cancer occurrence among a changing population as people move to or away from Connecticut. The population at risk at any given moment comprises current residents of Connecticut, but since residency may change and, in particular, new residents may be added to the population, the population being described is dynamic, not closed. Another example of a dynamic population might be that of a school, with new students entering each year and others leaving. An extreme example of a dynamic cohort would be the population of current U.S. presidents: whenever there is a new one, the previous one leaves the cohort, and whenever one leaves, a new one takes over; thus, the size of the population always remains constant at one.

In contrast to a dynamic cohort, a closed cohort always becomes smaller with passing time (Fig. 4–1). Investigators of a closed cohort will ideally attempt to track down cohort members if they leave the vicinity of the study. Members of a closed cohort constitute a group of people who remain members of the cohort even if they leave the area of the study. In a dynamic population that is defined geographically, however, people who leave the geographic boundaries of the study would not be followed.

Counting Disease Events

In cohort studies, epidemiologists usually calculate incidence rates or risks by dividing the number of new disease events (by *disease events*, we mean the number of disease onsets) by the appropriate denominator, based on the size of the population at risk. Usually, there are one or more categories of disease that are of special interest, and new cases of those diseases are counted. Occasionally, however, some disease onsets are excluded, even if they represent the disease under study.

One reason to exclude a disease event might be that it is not the first occurrence of the disease in that person. For example, suppose a woman develops cancer in one breast and later develops cancer in the other breast. In many studies, the second onset of breast cancer would not be counted as a new case, despite all biologic indications that it represents a separate cancer rather than the spread of the first cancer. Similarly, in many studies of myocardial infarction, only the first myocardial infarc-

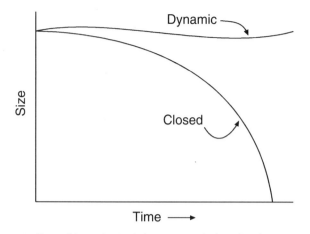

Figure 4–1. Size of hypothetical dynamic and closed cohorts over time.

tion is counted as a disease event and subsequent heart attacks are excluded. Why should investigators make this distinction between the first occurrence of a disease and subsequent occurrences? First, it may be difficult to distinguish between a new case of disease and a recurrence or exacerbation of an earlier case. Second, recurrent disease may have a different set of causes from the primary occurrence. If the investigator limits his or her interest to the first occurrence, all subsequent occurrences would be excluded, but there would also have to be a corresponding adjustment in the population at risk. Specifically, if only the first occurrence of disease is of interest, then any person who develops the disease is removed from the population at risk at the time that the disease develops. This procedure is consistent with the requirement that members of the population at risk must be eligible to develop the disease. If only the first occurrence is counted, people who develop the disease terminate their eligibility to acquire the disease at the point at which they develop disease.

If the epidemiologist is interested in measuring the total number of disease events, regardless of whether they are first or later occurrences, then a person who is in the cohort would remain as part of the population at risk even after getting the disease. In such an analysis, however, the first disease event would be counted just the same as a subsequent event and there would be no way to distinguish the occurrence of first versus later events. One way to make this distinction is to calculate separate occurrence measures for first and subsequent events. One could, for example, calculate the incidence rate of first events, second events, third events, and so forth. The population at risk for second events would be those who have had a first event. Upon having a first event, a person would leave the population at risk for a first event and enter the population at risk for a second event.

Another reason that a disease event might not be counted is that there was insufficient time for the disease to be related to an exposure. This issue is addressed below (see Exposure and Induction Time).

Measuring Incidence Rates or Risks

From a closed cohort we can estimate either a risk or an incidence rate to measure disease occurrence. Calculation of a risk is complicated by competing risks, discussed in Chapter 3. Because of competing risks, the population at risk will not remain constant in size over time, which means that some people will be removed from the population at risk before they have experienced the entire period of follow-up. Despite this problem, there are many cohort studies in which risks are estimated directly. Usually, the period of follow-up is short enough, or the competing risks are small enough in relation to the disease under study, that there is relatively little distortion in the risk estimates. In such studies, the risk in each cohort is calculated by dividing the number of new disease events by the total number of people being followed in the closed cohort. This approach was used to calculate the risk for cholera in Snow's analysis depicted in Table 4–1. Essentially the same approach was used in the study of vitamin A and birth defects described above, although the measure reported is the prevalence, rather than the risk, of birth defects.

It is problematic to measure risk directly in a dynamic cohort, where new people are added during the follow-up period. To get around this problem, one can take into account the amount of time that each person spends in the population at risk and calculate an incidence rate by dividing the number of new disease events by the amount of person-time experienced by the population at risk. The same approach could be applied to a closed cohort, thus addressing the problem of competing risks.

In the calculation of an incidence rate, the ideal situation is to have precise information on the amount of time that each person has been in the population at risk. Often, this time will be calculated for each person in terms of days at risk, although the final results may be expressed in terms of years after converting the units.

Cohort Study of X-Ray Fluoroscopy and Breast Cancer—An Example

The data in Table 3–6 are taken from a retrospective cohort study of radiation exposure and breast cancer. As part of their treatment for tuberculosis, many of the women received substantial doses of x-ray radiation for fluoroscopic monitoring of their lungs. Because the women were followed for highly variable lengths of time, it would not have been reasonable to calculate directly the risk of breast cancer; to do so requires a fixed length of follow-up for all people in a cohort. (They could have calculated the risk of breast cancer for segments of the follow-up time, using the life-table method described in Chapter 3.) Instead, the investigators measured the incidence rate of breast cancer among women with x-ray exposure. They compared this rate with the rate of breast cancer among women treated during the same period for tuberculosis but not with x-rays. The data in Table 3–6 show that the women who received x-ray exposure had nearly twice the incidence rate of breast cancer as the women who did not receive x-ray exposure.

Exposure and Induction Time

After the Second World War, the United States and Japan jointly undertook a cohort study of the populations of Hiroshima and Nagasaki who survived the atomic bomb blasts. These populations have been followed for decades, initially under the aegis of the Atomic Bomb Casualty Commission and later under its successor, the Radiation Effects Research Foundation. A category of outcome that has been of primary interest to the researchers has been cancer occurrence. Leukemia is one of the types of cancer that is substantially increased in incidence by ionizing radiation. Let us consider the survivors to constitute several closed cohorts, each corresponding to a different dose of ionizing radiation. The main factors that determined the dose of exposure were the distance from the epicenter of the blast and the shielding provided by the immediate environment, such as buildings, at the time of the blast.

Suppose that we wish to measure the incidence rate of leukemia among atomic bomb survivors who received a high dose of ionizing radiation and to compare this rate with the rate experienced by those who received little or no radiation exposure. The cohorts are defined at the time of the blasts, and their subsequent experience is tracked as part of the cohort study. Thus, we might consider that those who received a high dose of ionizing radiation immediately entered the population at risk for leukemia. The difficulty with beginning the follow-up immediately after the exposure is that it does not allow sufficient induction time for leukemia to develop as a result of the radiation exposure. For example, an exposed person who was diagnosed with leukemia 2 weeks after exposure is unlikely to have developed the disease as a consequence of the radiation exposure. After the exposure, disease does not occur until the induction period has passed (see Chapter 2). The induction period corresponds to the time that it takes for the causal mechanism to be completed by the action of the complementary component causes that act after radiation exposure. Suppose that the average time it takes before causal mechanisms that involve radiation are completed and leukemia occurs is 5 years and that few causal mechanisms are completed until 3 years have passed. After disease occurs, there is an additional interval, the latent period, during which disease exists but has not been diagnosed. It is important to keep both the induction period and the latent period in mind in the calculation of incidence rates. To measure the effect of radiation exposure most clearly, one should define the time period at risk for leukemia among exposed people in a way that allows for the induction time and perhaps for the latent period. Thus, it would make more sense to allow exposed people to enter the population at risk for leukemia only after a delay of at least 3 years, if we assume that any case occurring before that time could not plausibly be related to exposure.

Typically, the investigator cannot be sure what the induction time is for a given exposure and disease. In that case, it may be necessary to hypothesize various induction times and reanalyze the data under each separate hypothesis. Alternatively, there are statistical methods that estimate the most appropriate induction time.

Among exposed people, what happens to the person-time that is not related to exposure, under the hypothesis of a specific induction time? Consider the above example of studying the effect of radiation exposure from the atomic bomb blasts on the development of leukemia. If we hypothesize that no leukemia can occur as a result of the radiation until at least 3 years have elapsed since the blast, what happens to those first 3 years of follow-up for someone who was exposed? The question is akin to asking "How should we treat the experience of exposed people before they are exposed?" Although the induction time comes after exposure, it is a period during which the exposure does not have any effect and, thus, is like the time that comes before exposure. There are two reasonable options for dealing with this time: ignore it or combine it with the follow-up time of people who were never exposed.

Let us use the hypothetical data in Figure 4–2 as an example of how to calculate incidence rates for exposed and unexposed cohorts in a cohort study. Figure 4–2 depicts the follow-up time for 10 people, five exposed and five unexposed, who were followed for up to 20 years after a point exposure. There are three ways in which follow-up can end: (1) the person can be followed until the end of the follow-up period of 20 years; (2) the person can be lost to follow-up; (3) the person can get the disease. Those who are followed for the full 20 years are said to be withdrawn at the end of follow-up. Suppose that we calculated the incidence rate among exposed people during the 20 years following exposure. From the figure, we see that the follow-up times for the first five people are 12, 20, 15, 2, and 10 years, which add to 59 years. In this experience of 59 years, three disease events have occurred, for an incidence rate of 3 events per 59 years, or $3/59$ yr^{-1}. We might prefer to express this rate as 5.1 cases per 100 person-years, or $5.1/100$ yr^{-1}. For the unexposed group, the follow-up times are 20, 18, 20, 11, and 20 years, for a total of 89 years, and there was only one disease event, for a rate of $1/89$ yr^{-1}, or $1.1/100$ yr^{-1}.

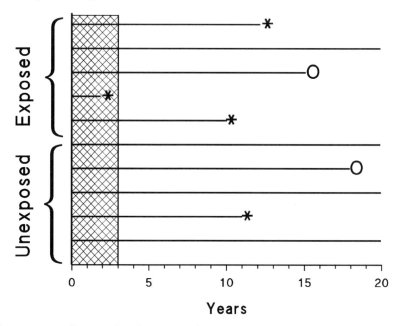

Figure 4–2. Follow-up data for 10 people in a hypothetical cohort study following five exposed people (top five lines) and five unexposed people (bottom five lines). The exposure was a point exposure that is hypothesized to have a minimum 3-year induction time (cross-hatched area) before any case of disease could result from it. * Disease event. ○, loss to follow-up.

The rate for the exposed group, however, does not take into account the 3-year induction period for exposure to have an effect. To take that into account, we would have to ignore the first 3 years of follow-up for the exposed group. Therefore, the follow-up times for the exposed cohort would be 9, 17, 12, 0, and 7 years, for a total of 45 years, with only two disease events occurring during this follow-up experience. The rate after taking into account the 3-year induction period would be $2/45 \text{ yr}^{-1}$, or $4.4/100 \text{ yr}^{-1}$. There is no reason to exclude the first 3 years of follow-up for the unexposed group, however, because there is no induction period among those who are not exposed. One might consider including the first 3 years of follow-up for each exposed person as unexposed experience because under the study hypothesis this experience is not related to exposure. If we did that, then the denominator of the rate for the unexposed would include 14 additional years of follow-up and one additional event, giving a rate of $2/103 \text{ yr}^{-1}$, or $1.9/100 \text{ yr}^{-1}$.

Retrospective Cohort Studies

A prospective cohort study is one in which the exposure information is recorded at the beginning of the follow-up and the period of time at risk for disease occurs during the conduct of the study. This is always the case with experiments and with many nonexperimental cohort studies.

Nevertheless, a cohort study is not always prospective: cohort studies can also be retrospective. In a *retrospective cohort study* (also known as *historical cohort studies*), the cohorts are identified from recorded information and the time during which they are at risk for disease occurred before the beginning of the study.

An outstanding example of a retrospective cohort study was conducted by Morrison and colleagues[9] of young women born in Florence in the fifteenth and sixteenth centuries. These women were enrolled in a dowry fund soon after they were born. The dowry fund was an insurance plan that would pay the family a sizeable return if an enrolled woman married. If the woman died or joined a convent first, the fund did not have to pay a dowry. The fund records contain the date of birth, date of investment, and date of dowry payment or death of 19,000 girls and women. More than 500 years after the first women were enrolled in the dowry fund, epidemiologists were able to use the fund records to chart waves of epidemic deaths from the plague and show how successive plague epidemics became milder over a period of 100 years. This retrospective cohort study, conducted centuries after the data were recorded, illustrates well that a cohort study need not be prospective.

Because a retrospective cohort study must rely on existing records, important information may be missing or otherwise unavailable. Nevertheless, when a retrospective cohort study is feasible, it offers the advantage of providing information that is usually much less costly than that from a prospective cohort study, and it may produce results much sooner because there is no need to wait for the disease to occur.

Tracing of Subjects

Cohort studies that span many years present a challenge with respect to maintaining contact with the cohort to ascertain disease events. Whether the study is retrospective or prospective, it is often difficult to locate people or their records many years after they have been enrolled into study cohorts. In prospective cohort studies, the investigator may contact study participants periodically to maintain current information on their location. Tracing subjects in cohort studies is a major component of their expense. If a large proportion of participants are lost to follow-up, the validity of the study may be threatened. Studies that trace fewer than about 60% of subjects are generally regarded with skepticism, but even follow-up of 70%, 80%, or more can be too low if the subjects lost to follow-up are lost for reasons related to both the exposure and the disease.

Special Exposure and General Population Cohorts

Cohort studies permit the epidemiologist to study many different disease end points at the same time. A mortality follow-up can be accomplished just as easily for all causes of death as for any specific cause.

Health surveillance for one disease end point can sometimes be expanded to include many or all end points without much additional work. A cohort study can provide a comprehensive picture of the health effect of a given exposure. Cohort studies that focus on people who share a particular exposure are called *special-exposure cohort studies*. Examples of special-exposure cohorts include occupational cohorts exposed to substances in the workplace; soldiers exposed to Agent Orange in Vietnam; residents of the Love Canal area of Niagara, New York, exposed to chemical wastes; Seventh Day Adventists exposed to vegetarian diets; and atomic bomb victims exposed to ionizing radiation. Each of these exposures is uncommon; therefore, it is usually more efficient to study them by identifying a specific cohort of people who have sustained that exposure and comparing their disease experience with that of a cohort of people who lack the exposure.

In contrast, common exposures are sometimes studied through cohort studies that survey a segment of the population identified initially without regard to exposure status. Such *general-population cohorts* typically focus on exposures that a substantial proportion of people have experienced. Otherwise, there would be too few people in the study who are exposed to the factors of interest. Once a general-population cohort is assembled, the cohort members can be classified according to smoking, alcoholic beverage consumption, diet, drug use, medical history, and many other factors of potential interest. The study described above of vitamin A intake in pregnant women and birth defects among their offspring[7] is an example of a general-population cohort study. No women in that study were selected because they had vitamin A exposure. Their exposure to vitamin A was determined after they were selected, during the interview. Although this was a general-population cohort study, a high level of vitamin A intake during pregnancy was not a common exposure. From Table 4–4, we can see that only 317 of the 22,058 women, or 1.4%, were in the highest category of vitamin A intake. Fortunately, the overall study population was large enough so that the vitamin A analysis was feasible; it would have been difficult to identify a special-exposure cohort of women who had a high intake of vitamin A during pregnancy.

In both special-exposure and general-population cohort studies, the investigator must classify study participants into the exposure categories that form the cohorts. This classification is easier for some exposures than for others. When the female offspring of women who took diethylstilbestrol were assembled for a special-exposure cohort study, defining their exposure was comparatively clear-cut, based on whether or not their mothers took diethylstilbestrol while they were pregnant.[10] For other exposures, however, such as second-hand smoke or dietary intake of saturated fat, nearly everyone is exposed to some extent; and the investigator studying such exposures must group people together according to their level of intake to form cohorts.

Case-Control Studies

The main drawback of conducting a cohort study is the necessity, in many situations, to obtain information on exposure and other variables from large populations in order to measure the risk or rate of disease. In many studies, however, only a tiny minority of those who are at risk for disease actually develop the disease. The case-control study aims at achieving the same goals as a cohort study but more efficiently, using sampling. Properly carried out, case-control studies provide information that mirrors what could be learned from a cohort study, usually at considerably less cost and time.

Case-control studies are best understood by considering as the starting point a *source population,* which represents a hypothetical study population in which a cohort study might have been conducted. The *source population* is the population that gives rise to the cases included in the study. If a cohort study were undertaken, we would define the exposed and unexposed cohorts (or several cohorts) and from these populations obtain denominators for the incidence rates or risks that would be calculated for each cohort. We would then identify the number of cases occurring in each cohort and calculate the risk or incidence rate for each. In a case-control study, the same cases are identified and classified as to whether they belong to the exposed or unexposed cohort. Instead of obtaining the denominators for the rates or risks, however, a control group is sampled from the entire source population that gives rise to the cases. Individuals in the control group are then classified into exposed and unexposed categories. The purpose of the control group is to determine the relative size of the exposed and unexposed components of the source population. Because the control group is used to estimate the distribution of exposure in the source population, the cardinal requirement of control selection is that the controls be sampled independently of exposure status.

Figure 4–3 illustrates the relation between a case-control study and the cohort study that it replaces. In the illustration, 25% of the 288 people in the source population are exposed. Suppose that the cases, illustrated at the right, arise during 1 year of follow-up. The rate of disease among exposed people would be 8 cases occurring in 72 person-years, for a rate of 0.111 cases per person-year. Among the 216 unexposed people, 8 additional cases arise during the 1 year of follow-up, for a rate of 0.037 cases per person-year. Thus, in this hypothetical example, the incidence rate among the exposed cohort is three times the rate among the unexposed cohort. Now consider what might happen if a case-control

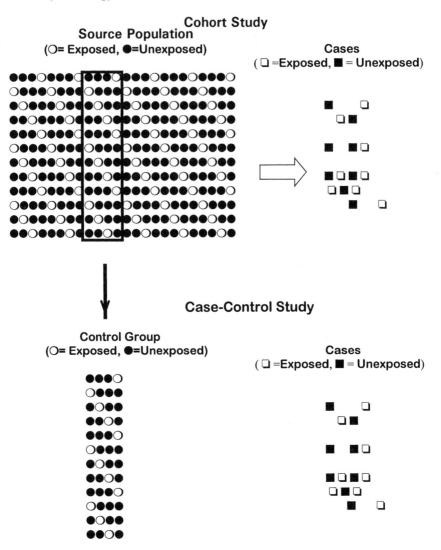

Figure 4–3. Schematic of a cohort study and a nested case-control study within the cohort showing how the control group is sampled from the source population.

study were conducted. The rectangle drawn around a portion of the source population represents a sample that might become the control group. It is essential that this sample be taken independently of the exposure. Among the 48 people in the control group, 12 are exposed. If the sample is taken independently of the exposure, the same proportion of controls will be exposed as the proportion of people (or person-time) exposed in the original source population. The same cases that were included in the cohort study are also included in the case-control study as the case group. We will shortly see how the data in the case-control study can be used to estimate the ratio of the incidence rates in the source population, giving the same result for the incidence rate ratio that the cohort study provides.

Nested Case-Control Studies

It is helpful to think of every case-control study as being nested, or conducted, within cohorts of exposed and unexposed people, as illustrated in Figure 4–3. Epidemiologists sometimes refer to specific case-control studies as *nested* case-control studies when the population within which the study is conducted is a well-defined cohort, but nearly any case-control study can be thought of as nested within some source population. In many instances, this population may be identifiable, for example, all residents of Rio de Janeiro during the year 2001; but in other instances, the members of the source population might be hard to identify.

In occupational epidemiology, a commonly used approach is to conduct a case-control study nested within an occupational cohort that has already been enumerated. The reason for conducting a case-control study even when a cohort can be enumerated is usually that more information is needed than is readily available from records and it would be too expensive to seek this information for everyone in the cohort. A nested case-control study is then more efficient. In such studies, the source population is easy to identify: it is the occupational cohort. A control group can be selected by sampling randomly from this source population.

As an example of a case-control study in which the source population is hard to identify, consider one in which the cases are patients treated for severe psoriasis at the Mayo Clinic. These patients come to the Mayo Clinic from all corners of the world. What is the specific source population that gives rise to these cases? To answer this question, we would have to know exactly who would go to the Mayo Clinic for severe psoriasis. Obviously, we cannot identify this population because many people in it do not know themselves that they would go to, or be referred to, the Mayo Clinic for severe psoriasis unless they actually developed it. Nevertheless, we can still imagine a population spread around the world that constitutes those people who would go to the Mayo Clinic if they developed severe psoriasis. It is this population in which the case-control study is nested and from which the control series would ideally be drawn. (In practice, one would likely draw the controls from other patients who attended the Mayo Clinic, who might constitute a 'proxy sample.') From this perspective, almost any case-control study can be thought of as nested within a source population, and a description of this population corresponds to eligibility criteria for both cases and controls.

Density Case-Control Study Design

There is more than one way to sample controls in a case-control study. One of the most common methods leads to a case-control study design using 'density-based sampling.' (The phrase comes from the term *incidence density*, which is sometimes used as a synonym for incidence rate.) Suppose that in a source population we have an exposed and an unexposed cohort, which we denote by the subscripts 1 and 0, respectively. During a given time period, the incidence rates for the exposed population would be

$$I_1 = \frac{a}{PT_1}$$

and, for the unexposed population,

$$I_0 = \frac{b}{PT_0}$$

where I_1 and I_0 are the incidence rates among exposed and unexposed, respectively; a and b are the respective numbers of exposed and unexposed people who developed the disease; and PT_1 and PT_0 are the respective amounts of person-time at risk for the exposed and the unexposed cohorts.

In a case-control study with density-based sampling, the control series provides an estimate of the proportion of the total person-time for exposed and unexposed cohorts in the source population. Suppose that the control series sampled from the source population contains c exposed people and d unexposed people. The aim is to select the control series so that the following ratios are equal, apart from statistical sampling error:

$$\frac{c}{d} = \frac{PT_1}{PT_0}$$

or, equivalently:

$$\frac{c}{PT_1} = \frac{d}{PT_0}$$

The ratios c/PT_1 and d/PT_0 are called the control sampling rates for the exposed and unexposed components of the source population. These sampling rates will be equal if the control sampling is conducted independently of exposure. If this goal is achieved, then the incidence rate ratio can be readily estimated from the case-control data as follows.

$$\frac{I_1}{I_0} = \frac{{}^a/_{PT_1}}{{}^b/_{PT_0}} = \frac{a}{b} \cdot \frac{PT_0}{PT_1} = \frac{a}{b} \cdot \frac{d}{c}$$

because

$$\frac{d}{c} = \frac{PT_0}{PT_1}$$

The quantity ad/bc, which in a case-control study provides an estimate of the incidence rate ratio, is called either the *cross-product ratio* or, more commonly, the *odds ratio*. Using the odds ratio in a case-control study, one can obtain a valid estimate of the incidence rate ratio in a population without having to obtain individual information on every person in the population.

What disadvantage is there in using a sample of the denominators rather than measuring the person-time experience for the entire source population? For one thing, sampling of the source population could lead to an inaccurate measure of the exposure distribution, giving rise to an incorrect estimate. Thus, a case-control study offers less statistical precision in estimating the incidence rate ratio than a cohort study of the same population. A loss in precision is to be expected whenever sampling is involved. This loss can be kept small if the number of controls selected per case is large. Furthermore, the loss is offset by the cost savings of not having to obtain information on everyone in the source population. The cost savings might allow the epidemiologist to enlarge the source population and, thus, obtain more cases, resulting in a better overall estimate of the incidence rate ratio, statistically and otherwise, than would be possible using the same expenditures to conduct a cohort study.

Defining the Source Population

The above discussion presumes that all people who develop the disease of interest in the source population are included as cases in the case-control study. Thus, the definition of the source population corresponds to the eligibility criteria for cases to enter the study. In theory, it is not necessary to include all cases occurring within an identifiable population, such as within a geographic boundary. The cases identified in a single clinic or treated by a single medical practitioner can be used for case-control studies. The corresponding source population for the cases treated in a clinic is all people who would attend that clinic and be recorded with the diagnosis of interest if they had the disease in question. It is important to specify "if they had the disease in question" because clinics serve different populations for different diseases, depending on referral patterns and the reputation of the clinic in specific specialty areas. Unfortunately, without a precisely identified source population, it may be difficult or impossible to select controls in an unbiased fashion.

Control Selection

In density case-control studies, the control series is sampled to represent the person-time distribution of exposure in the source population. If the sampling is conducted independently of the exposure, the case-control study can provide a valid estimate of the incidence rate ratio. Each control sampled will represent a certain amount of person-time experience. Thus, the probability of any given person in the source population being selected as a control should be proportional to his or her person-time contribution to the denominators of the incidence rates in the source population. For example, a person who is at risk of becoming a study case for 5 years should have a five times higher probability of being selected as a control than a person who is at risk for only 1 year.

For each person contributing time to the source population experience, the time that he or she is eligible to be selected as a control is the same time during which he or she is also eligible to become a case if the disease should occur. Thus, a person who has already developed the disease or has died is no longer eligible to be selected as a control. This rule corresponds to the treatment of subjects in cohort studies: every case that is tallied in the numerator of a cohort study contributes to the denominator of the rate until the time that the person becomes a case, when the contribution to the denominator ceases.

One way to implement control sampling according to the above guidelines is to choose controls from the unique set of people in the source population who are at risk of becoming a case at the precise time that each case is diagnosed. This set, which changes from one case to the next as people enter and leave the source population, is sometimes referred to as the *risk set* for the case. Risk-set sampling allows the investigator to sample controls so that each is selected in proportion to his or her time contribution to the person-time at risk.

A conceptually important feature of the selection of controls is their continuous eligibility to become cases if they should develop the disease. Suppose the study period spans 3 years, and that a given person free of disease in year 1 is selected as a control. The same person might go on to develop the disease in year 3, thus becoming a case. How is such a person treated in the analysis? If the disease is uncommon, it will matter little since a study is unlikely to have many subjects eligible to be both a case and a control; but the question is nevertheless of some theoretical interest. Since the person in question did develop disease during the study period, many investigators would be tempted to count the person as a case, not as a control. Recall, however, that if a cohort study were being conducted, each person who develops the disease would contribute not only to the numerator of the disease rate but also to the person-time experience counted in the denominator, until the time of disease onset. The control group in case-control studies is intended to provide estimates of the relative size of the denominators of the incidence rates for the compared groups. Therefore, each case in a case-control study should have been eligible to be a control before the time of disease onset; each control should be eligible to become a case as of the time of selection as a control. A person selected as a control who later develops the disease and is selected as a case should be included in the study both as a control and as a case.

As an extension of the previous point, a person selected as a control who remains in the study population at risk after selection should remain eligible to be selected once again as a control. Thus, although unlikely in typical studies, the same person may appear in the control group two or more times. Note, however, that including the same person at different times does not necessarily lead to exposure (or confounder) information being repeated because this information may change with time. For example, in a case-control study of an acute epidemic of intestinal illness, one might ask about food ingested within the previous day or days. If a contaminated food item was a cause of the illness for some cases, then the exposure status of a case or control chosen 5 days into the study might well differ from what it would have been 2 days into the study, when the subject might (also) have been included as a control.

Illustration of Case-Control Data

Consider again the data for the cohort study in Table 3–6. These data are shown again in Table 4–5 along with a hypothetical control series of 500 women who might have been selected from the two cohorts.

The ratio of the rates for the exposed and unexposed cohorts is $14.6/7.9 = 1.86$. Let us suppose that instead of conducting a cohort study, the investigators conducted a density case-control study by identifying all 56 breast cancer cases that occurred in the two cohorts and a control series of 500 women. The control series should be sampled from the person-time of the source population so that the exposure distribution of the controls sampled mirrors the exposure distribution of the person-time in the source population. Of the 47,027 person-years of experience in the combined exposed and unexposed cohorts, 28,010 (59.6%) are person-years of experience that relate to exposure. If the controls are sampled properly, we would expect that more or less 59.6% of them would be exposed and the remainder unexposed. If we happened to get just the proportion that we would expect to get on the average, we would have 298 exposed controls and 202 unexposed controls, as indicated in Table 4–5.

Table 4–5 shows the case and control series along with the full cohort data for comparison. In an actual case-control study, the data would

Table 4–5. Hypothetical case-control data drawn from a cohort study of breast cancer among women treated for tuberculosis with x-ray fluoroscopies and the full cohort data for comparison

	Radiation Exposure		
	Yes	No	Total
Breast cancer cases	41	15	56
(person-years)	(28,010)	(19,017)	(47,027)
Control series (people)	298	202	500
Rate (cases/10,000 person-years)	14.6	7.9	11.9

look like those in Table 4–6. Because there are two rows of data and two columns with four cell frequencies in the table (not counting the totals on the right), this type of table is often referred to as a 2 × 2 table. From these data, we can calculate the odds ratio to get an estimate of the incidence rate ratio.

$$\text{Odds ratio} = \frac{41 \times 202}{15 \times 298} = 1.85 = \text{Incidence rate ratio}$$

This result differs from the incidence rate ratio from the full cohort data by only a slight rounding error. Ordinarily we would expect to see additional error because the control group is a sample from the source population, and there may be some difference between the exposure distribution in the control series and the exposure distribution in the source population. In Chapter 7, we show how to take this sampling error into account.

Sources for Control Series

There are a number of options in case-control studies for selecting a control series: (1) population controls, (2) neighborhood controls, (3) random-digit dialing, (4) hospital- or clinic-based controls, and (5) dead people, among others.

Table 4–6. Case-control data alone from Table 4–5

	Radiation Exposure		
	Yes	No	Total
Breast cancer cases	41	15	56
Controls	298	202	500

Population controls

If the cases come from a precisely defined and identified population and the controls are sampled directly from this population, the study is said to be *population-based*. For a population-based case-control study, random sampling of controls may be feasible if a population register exists or can be compiled. When random sampling from the source population of cases is feasible, it is often the most desirable option.

Random sampling of controls does not necessarily mean that every person has an equal probability of being selected as a control. As explained above, if the aim is to estimate the incidence rate ratio, then we would employ density sampling, in which a person's control selection probability is proportional to the person's time at risk. For example, in a case-control study nested within an occupational cohort, workers on an employee roster will have been followed for varying lengths of time, and our random sampling scheme should reflect these varying times.

Neighborhood controls

If the source population cannot be enumerated, it may be possible to select controls by sampling residences in some systematic fashion. If a geographic roster of residences is not available, some scheme must be devised to sample residences without enumerating them all. Often, matching is employed as a convenience: after a case is identified, one or more controls who reside in the same neighborhood as that case are identified and recruited into the study.

Random-digit dialing

If case eligibility includes residence in a house that has a telephone, randomly calling telephone numbers simulates a random sample of the source population. Random-digit dialing offers the advantage of approaching all households in a designated area, even those with unlisted telephone numbers, through a simple telephone call. The method poses a few challenges, however.

First, even if the investigator can implement a sampling method so that every telephone has the same probability of being called, there will not necessarily be the same probability of contacting each eligible control subject, because households vary in the number of people who reside in them and the amount of time someone is at home. Second, making contact with a household may require many calls at various times of day and various days of the week. Third, it may be challenging to distinguish business from residential telephone numbers, a distinction that affects calculating the proportion of nonresponders. Other problems include answering machines and households with multiple telephone numbers, a rapidly increasing phenomenon. The increase in telemarketing in the United States and the availability of caller identification has further compromised response rates to "cold-calling." To obtain a control subject meeting specific eligibility characteristics can require dozens of telephone calls on the average. As the number of household telephone lines continues to increase and to vary from household to household, random-digit dialing will become less useful as a method for sampling controls from the source population, because it will tend to oversample people from households with multiple telephone lines.

Hospital- or clinic-based controls
In hospital- or clinic-based case-control studies, the source population represents a group of people who would be treated in a given clinic or hospital if they developed the disease in question. This population may be hard to identify. If the hospitals or clinics that provide the cases for the study treat only a small proportion of those in the geographic area, then referral patterns to the hospital or clinic are important to take into account in the sampling of controls. For these studies, it is appropriate to consider drawing a control series comprising patients from the same hospitals or clinics as the cases. It is important to keep in mind that the source population does not correspond to the population of the geographic area, but only to the people who "feed" the hospital or clinic with the cases of the disease under study. Other patients treated at the same hospitals or clinics as the cases will constitute a sample, albeit not a random one, of this source population.

The major problem with any nonrandom sampling of controls is the possibility that they are not selected independently of exposure in the source population. Patients hospitalized with other diseases at the same hospitals, for example, may not have the same exposure distribution as the entire source population, either because exposed people are more or less likely than nonexposed people to be hospitalized for the control diseases if they develop them or because the exposure may cause or prevent these control diseases in the first place. For example, suppose the study aims at evaluating the relation between tobacco smoking and leukemia. If controls are people hospitalized with other conditions, many of them will have been hospitalized for conditions that are caused by smoking. A variety of other cancers, as well as cardiovascular diseases and respiratory diseases, are related to smoking. Thus, a series of people hospitalized for diseases other than leukemia would include more smokers than the source population from which they came. One approach to this problem is to exclude any diagnosis from the control series that is likely to be related to the exposure. For example, in the imagined study of smoking and leukemia, one could exclude from the control series anyone who was hospitalized with a disease thought to be related to smoking. This approach may lead to the exclusion of many diagnostic categories, but even a few diagnostic categories should suffice to find enough control subjects.

It is risky, however, to reduce the control eligibility criteria to a single diagnosis. Using a variety of diagnoses has the advantage of diluting any bias that might result from including a specific diagnostic group that is in fact related to the exposure. For any diagnostic category that is excluded, the exclusion criterion should be applied only with regard to the cause of the hospitalization used to identify the study subject, rather than to any previous hospitalization. A person who was hospitalized because of a traumatic injury and is thus eligible to be a control would not be excluded if he or she had previously been hospitalized for cardiovascular disease. The reason is that the source population includes people who have had cardiovascular disease, and they must also be included in the control series.

Dead people

Dead people are not in the source population for cases, since death will preclude the occurrence of any further disease. The main argument for choosing dead controls is that if the cases are dead from their disease, choosing dead controls will enhance comparability. While certain types of comparability are important, choosing dead controls will misrepresent the exposure distribution in the source population if the exposure causes or prevents death in a substantial number of people or if it is associated with another factor that does. If interviews are needed and some cases are dead, it will be necessary to use proxy respondents for the dead cases. To enhance comparability of information while avoiding the problems of taking dead controls, proxy respondents can also be used for live controls who are matched to dead cases. In some situations, however, it may be reasonable to choose dead controls, despite the fact that they are not part of the source population. The justification for doing so is simply convenience. For example, a study may be based entirely on a series of deaths.

What is the theoretical justification for including controls who are not members of the source population for cases? If a control series can provide the same exposure distribution as a control series that would have been sampled directly from the source population, then it is valid. Consider a case-control study examining the relation between ABO blood type and female breast cancer. Could such a study have a control series comprising the brothers of the female cases? The brothers of the cases are not part of the source population. Nevertheless, the distribution of ABO blood type among the brothers should be identical to the distribution among the source population of women who might have been included as cases, because ABO blood type is not related to sex. Similarly, if a series of dead controls would provide the same exposure distribution as the source population, it is a reasonable control series to use. When we use a control series that is not part of the source population to estimate the exposure distribution in the source population, it is described as *proxy sampling*. When clinic patients with disease diagnoses different

---

Is representativeness important?

Some textbooks claim that cases should be representative of all persons with the disease and that controls should be representative of the entire nondiseased population. Such advice can be misleading. In fact, cases can be defined in any way that the investigator wishes and need not be representative of all cases. Thus, older cases, female cases, severe cases, or any clinical subset of cases could be studied. These groups are not representative of all cases but would be allowable as case definitions. Indeed, any type of case that could be used as the disease event in a cohort study could also be used to define the case series in a case-control study.

  The case definition will implicitly define the source population for cases, from which the controls should be drawn. It is this source population for the cases that the controls should represent, not the entire nondiseased population.

---

from that of the cases are used as controls, that may also be proxy sampling, if those control patients would not have come to the same clinic if they had been diagnosed with the disease that the cases have.

Case-Cohort Study Design

Recall that in density case-control studies, the control series represents the person-time distribution of exposure in the source population. That representativeness is achieved by sampling controls in such a way that the probability that any person in the source population is selected as a control is proportional to his or her person-time contribution to the incidence rates in the source population. In contrast, the *case-cohort study* is a case-control study in which every person in the source population has the same chance of being included as a control, regardless of how much time that person has contributed to the person-time experience of the cohort. This is a reasonable way to conduct a case-control study if people in the source population have been followed for the same length of time. With this type of sampling, each control participant represents a fraction of the total number of people in the source population, rather than a fraction of the total person-time. The odds ratio, calculated just as in a density case-control study, has a slightly different interpretation in a case-cohort study.

$$\text{Odds ratio} = \frac{ad}{bc}$$

Because c and d, the number of exposed and unexposed controls, respectively, are sampled from the list of all cohort members rather than from the person-time experience in the source population, the odds ratio in a case-cohort study is an estimate of the risk ratio rather than the rate ratio. It is as if we had calculated risks in a cohort rather than taking into account the time that each person is at risk during the follow-up period. Of course, if risks are small, then the risk ratio is approximately equal to the incidence rate ratio, so in many instances there may be little difference between the result from a case-cohort study and the result from a density case-control study.

If the proportion of subjects that is sampled and becomes part of the control series is known, it is possible to estimate the actual size of the cohorts being followed and the separate risks for the exposed and unexposed cohorts. Usually, this sampling proportion is not known, in which case the actual risks cannot be calculated. As long as the controls are sampled independently of the exposure, however, the odds ratio will still be a valid estimate of the risk ratio, just as the odds ratio in a density case-control study is an estimate of the incidence rate ratio.

The main reason that a case-cohort study is conducted instead of a density case-control study is convenience. Data that allow risk-set sampling may not be available, for example. Furthermore, the investigators may intend to study several diseases. In risk-set sampling, each control must be sampled from the risk set (the set of people in the source population who are at risk for disease at that time) for each case. The definition of the risk set changes for each case because the identity of the risk set is related to the timing of the case. If several diseases are to be studied, each one would require its own control group to maintain risk-set sampling. Control sampling for a case-cohort study, however, requires just a single sample of people from the roster of people who constitute the cohort. The same control group could be used to compare with various case series, just as the same denominators for calculating risks would be used to calculate the risk for various diseases in the cohort. This approach can therefore be considerably more convenient than density sampling.

In a case-cohort study, a person who is selected as a control may also be a case. (The same possibility exists in a density case-control study.) This possibility may seem bothersome; some epidemiologists take pains to avoid the possibility that a control subject might have even an undetected stage of the disease under study. Nevertheless, there is no theoretical difficulty with a control participant also being a case. To understand why, keep in mind that the control series in a case-cohort study is a sample of the entire list of people in the exposed and unexposed cohorts. If we did not sample at all but included the entire list, we would have a cohort study from which we could directly calculate risks for exposed and unexposed groups. In a risk calculation, every person in the numerator (that is, every case) is also a person in the denominator (a person in the source population). Thus, some people appear in both the numerator and the denominator of a risk. This situation is analogous to the possibility that a person who is sampled as a control subject in a case-cohort study might be included as a case. If one thinks of the control series as being a sample of the exposed and unexposed cohorts at the start of follow-up, one can see that the control sampling represents people who were free of disease, because everyone at the start of follow-up in a cohort study is free of disease. It is only later that disease develops in some of these people, who then become cases. These parallels in thinking between case-control and cohort studies help to clarify the principles of control selection and illustrate the importance of viewing case-control studies simply as cohort studies with sampled denominators.

Illustration of Case-Cohort Data

Consider the data in Table 4–1 describing John Snow's natural experiment. Let us imagine that he had conducted a case-cohort study instead, with a sample of 10,000 controls selected from the source population of the London neighborhoods that he was investigating. If the control series had the same distribution by water company that the entire population in Table 4–1 had, the data might resemble the 2 × 2 Table 4–7. We would take the odds ratio from these hypothetical case-cohort data as follows:

$$\text{Odds ratio} = \frac{4093 \times 3946}{461 \times 6054} = 5.79 = \text{Risk ratio}$$

This result is essentially the same value that Snow obtained from his natural-experiment cohort study. In this hypothetical case-cohort study, 10,000 controls were included, instead of the 440,000 people Snow included in the full cohort-study comparison. If Snow had to determine the exposure status of every person in the population, it would have been much easier to conduct the case-cohort study and simply sample from the source population. As it happened, Snow derived his exposure distribution by estimating the population of water company customers from business records, making it unnecessary to obtain information on each person. He did have to ascertain the exposure status of each case, however.

Table 4–7. Hypothetical case-cohort data for John Snow's natural experiment

	Water Company	
	Southwark and Vauxhall	**Lambeth**
Cholera deaths	4093	461
Controls	6054	3946

The rare disease assumption

It has been claimed that the odds ratio from a case-control study estimates the incidence rate ratio or the risk ratio only if the disease is
rare. The reason for this belief relates to the strategy used for sampling
controls. For example, in a case-cohort study, controls are sampled
from the initial roster of all subjects, a strategy that provides a valid
estimate of the risk ratio whether disease is common or rare. If controls were instead sampled from those who, at the end of the follow-
up, remained free of disease, the odds ratio would overestimate the
risk ratio for a positive exposure–disease relation because the exposure proportion among those remaining free of disease at the end of
follow-up would be smaller than the exposure proportion among
those starting their follow-up. If disease were rare, however, the odds
ratio after using this sampling strategy would be a reasonable estimate
of the risk ratio. In density case-control studies or case-cohort studies,
there is no need for any rare disease assumption for the odds ratio to
be a valid estimate of the incidence rate ratio or the risk ratio,
respectively.

Prospective and Retrospective Case-Control Studies

Case-control studies, like cohort studies, can also be either prospective
or retrospective. In a retrospective case-control study, cases have already
occurred when the study begins; there is no waiting for new cases to
occur. In a prospective case-control study, the investigator must wait,
just as in a prospective cohort study, for new cases to occur.

Case-Crossover Studies

In recent years, many variants of case-control studies have been described. One that is compelling in its simplicity and elegance is the case-
crossover study, which is a case-control analogue of the crossover study.
A *crossover study* is an experimental study in which two (or more) interventions are compared, with each study participant acting as his or her
own control. Each subject receives both interventions in a random sequence, with some time interval between them so that the outcome can
be measured after each intervention. A crossover study thus requires
that the effect period of the intervention is short enough so that it does
not persist into the time period during which the next treatment is
administered.

The *case-crossover study,* first proposed by Maclure,[11] is a case-control
version of the crossover study. All subjects in a case-crossover study are
cases. The control series in a case-crossover study does not comprise a
different set of people but, rather, a sample of the time experience of the
cases before they developed disease. First, a study hypothesis is defined

---

Cohort/case-control studies versus prospective/retrospective studies

Early descriptions often referred to cohort studies as prospective studies and to case-control studies as retrospective studies. We now reserve the terms *prospective* and *retrospective* to refer to the timing of the information and events of the study, and we use the term *case-control* to describe studies in which the source population is sampled rather than ascertained in its entirety, as in a cohort study. The early descriptions carried the implication that retrospective studies were less valid than prospective studies, an idea that lingers. It is still commonly thought that case-control studies are less valid than cohort studies. The truth is that validity issues can affect either cohort or case-control studies, whether they are prospective or retrospective. Nevertheless, there is no reason to discount a study simply because it is a case-control study (or a retrospective study). Case-control studies represent a high achievement of modern epidemiology, and if conducted well, they can reach the highest standards of validity.

---

in relation to a specific exposure that causes the disease within a specified time period. Each case is considered exposed or unexposed according to the time relation specified in the hypothesis. Maclure[11] used the example of sexual intercourse causing myocardial infarction within 1 hour. Cases would be a series of people who have had a myocardial infarction. Each case would be classified as exposed if he or she had sexual intercourse within the hour preceding the myocardial infarction. Otherwise, the case would be classified as unexposed.

So far, this process differs little from what might be done for any case-control study. The key difference comes in obtaining the control "series." Instead of obtaining information from other people, in the case-crossover study, the control information is obtained from the cases themselves. In the example of sexual intercourse and myocardial infarction, the average frequency of sexual intercourse would be ascertained for each case during a period, say 1 year, before the myocardial infarction occurred. Under the study hypothesis, after each instance of sexual intercourse, the risk of myocardial infarction during the following hour is elevated, and that hour is considered exposed person-time. All other time would be considered unexposed. If a person had sexual intercourse once per week, then 1 hour per week would be considered exposed and the remaining 167 hours would be considered unexposed. Such a calculation can be performed for each case, and from the distribution of these hours within the experience of each case, the incidence rate ratio of myocardial infarction after sexual intercourse, in relation to the incidence rate at other times, can be estimated. The information for the study is obtainable in its entirety from a series of cases.

Only certain types of study question can be studied with a case-crossover design. The exposure must be something that varies from time to time within a person. One cannot study the effect of blood type in a case-crossover study. One can study whether coffee drinking triggers an asthma attack within a short time, however, because coffee is consumed intermittently. Indeed, it is convenient to think of the case-crossover study as evaluating exposures that trigger a short-term effect. In addition, the disease must have an abrupt onset. One could not study causes of multiple sclerosis in a case-crossover study, but one could study whether an automobile driver who is talking on a telephone is at higher risk of having a collision. Finally, the effect of the exposure must be brief. If the exposure had a long effect, then it would not be possible to relate the disease to a particular episode of exposure. How short is brief? The duration of the exposure effect should be shorter than the typical interval between episodes of exposure so that the effect of exposure is gone before the next episode of exposure occurs.

Is a case-crossover study a cohort study or a case-control study?

A case-crossover study uses the previous experience of the cases as a substitute for a control series, to estimate the person-time distribution in the source population. One way that it differs from a conventional case-control study is that the control information is not a distribution of control subjects, which is basically a frequency distribution of people by exposure category, but rather a distribution of the person-time experienced by the cases. In that regard, it resembles more closely a cohort study that measures incidence rates than it does a typical case-control study. Indeed, because the data in a case-crossover study involve cases and person-time, case-crossover studies are often analyzed using methods designed for cohort studies rather than case-control studies. So should we consider them to be cohort studies rather than case-control studies? It is certainly reasonable to view them as a restricted type of cohort study. Nevertheless, they clearly resemble case-control studies in that there is sampling of the source population experience, and as a result of the sampling, one can calculate only rate ratios, not rates or rate differences. In this way, case-crossover studies occupy a middle ground between cohort and case-control studies. Because there is sampling rather than complete enumeration of the source population experience, however, it does have the key characteristic of a case-control study.

Cross-Sectional versus Longitudinal Studies

All of the study types described thus far in this chapter would be described as *longitudinal* studies. In epidemiology, a study is considered to be longitudinal if the information obtained pertains to more than one point in time. Implicit in a longitudinal study is the universal premise that the causal action of an exposure comes before the subsequent development of disease as a consequence of that exposure. This concept is integral to the thinking involved in following cohorts over time or in sampling from the person-time at risk based on earlier exposure status. All cohort studies and most case-control studies rely on data in which exposure information refers to an earlier time than that of disease occurrence, making the study longitudinal.

Occasionally, epidemiologists conduct cross-sectional studies, in which all of the information refers to the same point in time. These studies are basically "snapshots" of the population status with respect to disease or exposure variables, or both, at a specific point in time. A population survey, such as the decennial census in the United States, is a cross-sectional study that not only attempts to enumerate the population but also assesses the prevalence of various characteristics. Similar surveys are conducted frequently to sample opinions, but they might also be used to measure disease prevalence or even to assess the relation between disease prevalence and possible exposures.

A cross-sectional study cannot measure disease incidence, because either risk or rate calculations require information across a time period. Nevertheless, cross-sectional studies can assess disease prevalence. It is possible to use cross-sectional data for a case-control study if the study includes prevalent cases and uses concurrent information about exposure. A case-control study that is based on prevalent cases, rather than new cases, will not necessarily provide information about the causes of disease. Because the cases in such a study are those who have the disease at a given point in time, the study is more heavily weighted with cases of long duration than any series of incident cases would be. A person who died soon after onset of disease, for example, would count as an incident case but likely would not be included as a case in a prevalence survey, because the disease duration is so brief.

Sometimes cross-sectional information is used because it is considered a good proxy for longitudinal data. For example, an investigator might wish to know how much supplemental vitamin E was consumed 10 years in the past. Since no written record of this exposure is likely to exist, the basic choices are to ask people to recall how much supplemental vitamin E they consumed in the past or to find out how much they consume now. Recall of past use is likely to be hazy, whereas current consumption can be determined accurately. In some situations, accurate current information may be a better proxy for the actual consumption 10 years earlier than the hazy recollections of that past consumption. Current consumption may be cross-sectional, but it would be used as a proxy for exposure in the past. Another example would be blood type: because it remains constant, cross-sectional information on blood type is a perfect proxy for past information about blood type. In this way, cross-sectional studies can sometimes be nearly as informative as longitudinal studies with respect to causal hypotheses.

Comparison of Cohort and Case-Control Studies

It may be helpful to summarize some of the key characteristics of cohort and case-control studies. The primary difference is that a cohort study involves complete enumeration of the denominator (people or person-time) of the disease measure, whereas case-control studies sample from the denominator. As a result, case-control studies provide estimates only of ratio measures of effect, whereas cohort studies provide estimates of disease rates and risks for each cohort, which can then be compared by taking differences or ratios. Case-control studies can be thought of simply as modified cohort studies, with sampling of the source population being the essential modification.

Consistent with this theme is the idea that many issues that apply to cohort studies apply to case-control studies in the same way. For example, if a person gets disease, that person no longer contributes time at risk to the denominator of a rate in a cohort study. Analogously, in a density case-control study, a person who gets disease is, from that point of time forward, no longer eligible to be sampled as a control. Another example of the parallels between cohort studies and case-control studies is the classification of studies into prospective and retrospective types.

Case-control studies are more efficient than cohort studies in the sense that the cost of the information they provide is often much lower. With a cohort study, it is often convenient to study many different disease outcomes in relation to a given exposure. With a case-control study, it is often convenient to study many different exposures in relation to a single disease. This contrast, however, is not absolute. In many cohort studies, a variety of exposures can be studied in relation to the disease(s) of interest. Likewise, in many case-control studies, the case series can be expanded to include more than one disease category, which in effect leads to several parallel case-control studies conducted within the same source population. These characteristics are summarized in Table 4–8.

Table 4–8. Comparison of the characteristics of cohort and case-control studies

Cohort Study	Case-Control Study
Complete source population denominator experience tallied	Sampling from source population
Can calculate incidence rates or risks and their differences and ratios	Can usually calculate only the ratio of incidence rates or risks
Usually very expensive	Usually less expensive
Convenient for studying many diseases	Convenient for studying many exposures
Can be prospective or retrospective	Can be prospective or retrospective

Questions

1. During the second half of the twentieth century, there was a sharp increase in hysterectomy procedures in the United States. Concurrent with that trend, there was an epidemic of endometrial cancer that has been attributed to widespread use of replacement estrogens among menopausal women. The epidemic of endometrial cancer was not immediately evident, however, in data on endometrial cancer rates compiled from cancer registries. Devise a hypothesis based on considerations of the population at risk for endometrial cancer that might explain why the epidemic went unnoticed.
2. What is the purpose of randomization in an experiment? How is the same goal achieved in nonexperimental studies?
3. When cancer incidence rates are calculated for the population covered by a cancer registry, the usual approach is to take the number of new cases of cancer and divide by the person-time contributed by the population covered by the registry. Person-time is calculated as the size of the population, from census data, multiplied by the time period. This calculation leads to an underestimate of the incidence rate in the population at risk. Explain.
4. In the calculations of rates for the data in Figure 4–2, the rate in the exposed group declined after taking the induction period into account. If exposure does cause disease, would you expect that the rate in exposed people would increase, decrease, or stay the same after taking into account an appropriate induction period?
5. If a person already has disease, can that person be selected as a control in a case-control study of that disease?
6. If a person has already been selected as a control in a case-control study and then later during the study period develops the disease being studied, should the person be kept in the study as (1) a case, (2) a control, (3) both, or (4) neither?
7. In case-cohort sampling, a single control group can be compared with various case groups in a set of case-control comparisons because the control sampling depends on the identity of the cohorts and has nothing to do with the cases. Analogously, the denominators of risk for a set of several different diseases occurring in the cohort would have the same denominator. Risk-set sampling, in contrast, requires that the investigator identify the risk set for each case; thus, the sample of controls will be different for each disease studied. If the analogy holds, this observation would imply that the denominators of incidence rates differ when calculating the rates for different diseases in the same cohort. Is that true? If not, why not? If so, why should the denominators for the risks not change no matter what disease is studied whereas the denominators for the rates change from studying one disease to another?
8. Explain why it would not be possible to study the effect of cigarette smoking on lung cancer in a case-crossover study but why it would

be possible to study the effect of cigarette smoking on sudden death from arrhythmia using that design.

9. Some case-control studies are conducted by sampling controls from those people who remain free of disease after the period of risk (such as an epidemic period) has ended. Demonstrate why, with this sampling strategy, the odds ratio will tend to be an overestimate of the risk ratio.

10. Often, the diagnosis of disease is taken as the disease onset. Many diseases, such as cancer, rheumatoid arthritis, and schizophrenia, may have been present in an earlier, undiagnosed form for a considerable time before the diagnosis. Suppose you are conducting a case-control study of a cancer. If it were possible, would it be preferable to exclude people with undetected cancer from the control series?

References

1. Last, JM: *A Dictionary of Epidemiology,* 3rd ed. New York: Oxford University Press, 1995.
2. Snow, J. *On the Mode of Communication of Cholera,* 2nd ed. London: John Churchill, 1860. (Facsimile of 1936 reprinted edition by Hafner, New York, 1965.)
3. Kinloch-de Loes, S, Hirschel, BJ, Hoen, B, et al: Controlled trial of zidovudine in primary human immunodeficiency virus infection. *N Engl J Med* 1995;333:408–413.
4. Francis, TF, Korns, RF, Voight, RB, et al: An evaluation of the 1954 poliomyelitis vaccine trials. *Am J Public Health* 1955;45(Suppl.):1–63.
5. Bang, AT, Bang, RA, Baitule, SB, et al: Effect of home-based neonatal care and management of sepsis on neonatal mortality: field trial in rural India. *Lancet* 1999;354:1955–1961.
6. Milunsky, A, Jick, H, Jick, SS, et al: Multivitamin/folic acid supplementation in early pregnancy reduces the prevalence of neural tube defects. *JAMA* 1989;262:2847–2852.
7. Rothman, KJ, Moore, LL, Singer, MR, et al: Teratogenicity of high vitamin A intake. *N Engl J Med* 1995;333:1369–1373.
8. Dawber, TR, Moore, FE, Mann, GV: Coronary heart disease in the Framingham study. *Am J Public Health* 1957;47:4–24.
9. Morrison, AS, Kirshner, J, Molho, A: Epidemics in renaissance Florence. *Am J Public Health* 1985;75:528–535.
10. Labarthe, D, Adam, E, Noller, KL, et al: Design and preliminary observations of National Cooperative Diethylstilbestrol Adenosis (DESAD) Project. *Obstet Gynecol* 1978;4:453–458.
11. Maclure, M: The case-crossover design: a method for studying transient effects on the risk of acute events. *Am J Epidemiol* 1991;133:144–153.

5

Biases in Study Design

Two broad types of error afflict epidemiologic studies: *random error* and *systematic error*. In designing a study, an epidemiologist attempts to reduce both sources of error. In interpreting a study, a reader ought to be aware of both types of error and how they have been addressed.

What exactly do we mean by error in a study? In Chapter 4, we began by stating that an epidemiologic study can be viewed as an attempt to obtain an epidemiologic measure. The object of measurement could be a rate or a risk, but it typically is a measure of effect, such as an incidence rate ratio. Suppose a study is conducted to measure the ratio of the incidence rate of Alzheimer's disease among those who are physically active compared with those who are physically inactive. We can imagine that there is a correct value for the incidence rate ratio. A given study will produce an estimate of this correct value. If the study estimates a value of the incidence rate ratio that is close to the correct value, we would consider the study to be accurate, which is to say that it has little error. Conversely, a study estimate that differs considerably from the correct value is inaccurate. Unfortunately, we can never know the correct value for the rate ratio for Alzheimer's disease among physically active people compared with the physically inactive, or for any other measure that we try to estimate; all we can ever know is the value of the estimates from a study. Because the correct values are unknown, we cannot determine the actual amount of error in any given study. Nevertheless, epidemiologists can still take steps in the design and analysis of studies to reduce errors. Furthermore, as readers, we can look for features in the design and analysis of a study that might either contribute to or prevent errors.

In this chapter, we focus on systematic error. (Random error will be discussed in Chapter 6, which deals with statistical issues in epidemiologic research.) Another term for systematic error is *bias*. Bias can refer to an attitude on the part of the investigator, but it is also used to describe any systematic error in a study. A study can be biased because of the way in which the subjects have been selected, the way the study variables are measured, or some confounding factor that is not completely controlled.

There is a simple way to distinguish random errors from systematic errors. Imagine that a given study could be increased in size until it was infinitely large. There are some errors that would be reduced to zero if a study became infinitely large; these are the random errors. Other errors are not affected by increasing the size of the study. Errors that remain even in an infinitely large study are the systematic errors (Fig. 5–1).

To see the difference between systematic errors and random errors, consider the following example. Suppose your task is to determine the average height of women in the city of Centerville, which has a population of 500,000 women. To conduct this work, you are supplied with an official measuring tape. You might decide to measure the height of 100 women sampled randomly from the population of all women in the city. You can use the average of the 100 measurements as an estimate of the average height of women in Centerville. What sources of error affect your estimate? A measuring tape will give different readings depending on how it is held, how it is read, the time of day the measurement is taken, and who is taking the measurement. Some of these errors, such as how the measuring tape is held during a given measurement, may be random. That is, some of these errors will sometimes lead to a reading that is too high and sometimes to a reading that is too low, but on the average, readings will not tend to be either too high or too low. If the

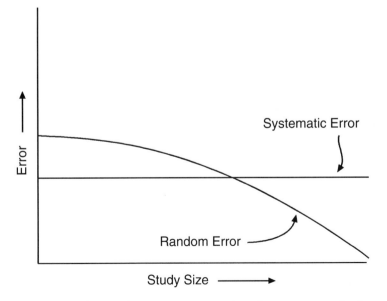

Figure 5–1. Relation of systematic error and random error to study size.

sample of 100 were increased to 1000 or to 10,000 women, the effect of these random errors would become less important because the greater number of measurements would ensure that the discrepancy between the average measured height for women in the sample and the height of all women in Centerville would be close to zero. There are other errors, however, that would not be affected by increasing the number of women measured. Suppose that the official tape used in the measurements was a cloth tape that had been laundered before the project began. Unknown to anyone, the laundering shrank the tape. Consequently, the height estimates derived from using the shrunken tape would tend to be high by an amount that depends on the amount of shrinkage. This systematic error cannot be reduced by taking more measurements with the same shrunken tape. Similarly, any defect in the measuring technique, such as a tendency to hold the tape crookedly, will also lead to measurements that are systematically wrong and would not be offset by increasing the number of subjects.

Sources of Bias in Epidemiologic Studies

Error can creep into epidemiologic studies from myriad directions. Although many types of specific bias have been described, it is helpful to classify bias into three broad categories: selection bias, information bias, and confounding.

Selection Bias

Selection bias is a systematic error in a study that stems from the procedures used to select subjects and from factors that influence study participation. It comes about when the association between exposure and disease differs for those who participate and those who do not participate in the study. Because the association between exposure and disease among nonparticipants is usually unknown, the presence of selection bias must usually be inferred, rather than observed.

Suppose that a new screening test was devised to detect colon cancer and that this test was offered to a community in a pilot evaluation. Later, the efficacy of the test was assessed by comparing the incidence rate of colon cancer among those who volunteered to be tested with the incidence rate among community residents who were not tested. We would suspect that such a comparison would suffer from selection bias. At issue is whether we might expect any difference in colon cancer incidence between these two groups regardless of whether the screening test had any effect. Very likely, there would be a difference: people who volunteer for cancer screening are generally more health-conscious than those who do not volunteer, and people who are more health-conscious may have a diet that lowers the risk of colon cancer. If so, then those who volunteer for screening might be expected to have a lower rate of colon cancer for reasons that do not result from the screening. This difference would be superimposed on any effect of the screening and represent a bias in assessing the screening effect.

Another possibility is that some of those who volunteer for screening may volunteer because they are especially worried about their colon cancer risk. They might, for example, have a family history of colon cancer. Thus, some volunteers may be at lower risk than non-volunteers, and other volunteers may be at a higher risk than nonvolunteers. These biases would tend to counteract one another, but because neither one is easy to quantify, the net bias would be unknown. Concern about selection bias has been the main reason why the efficacy of many screening procedures is evaluated by randomized trials. Although a randomized trial is much more cumbersome and expensive than a cohort study, the randomization assures that the groups are comparable if the study is reasonably large.

The selection bias in the above example arises from self-selection, because the study subjects selected themselves to be screened. Selection bias can also arise from choices made more directly by the investigator. For example, many studies of worker health have compared the death rate among workers in a specific job with that among the general population. This comparison is biased because the general population contains many people who cannot work because of ill health. Consequently, overall death rates for workers are often substantially lower than those for the general population, and any direct comparison of the two groups is biased. This selection bias is often referred to as the *healthy worker effect.* One way to avert the bias would be to compare the workers in a specific job with workers in other jobs that differ in occupational exposures or hazards. If all subjects involved in the comparison are workers, the investigator can thus avoid bias from the healthy worker effect.

Table 5–1 shows how the healthy worker effect comes about. If the mortality rate of an exposed group of workers at a specific plant is compared with that of the general population (the total column in Table 5–1), their overall mortality rate appears much lower; in this hypothetical example, their overall mortality rate is 5/7, or 71% of the rate in the general population. The general population, however, comprises two groups: a majority that is healthy enough to work and a minority that is too ill to work. The latter group is included among the nonworkers in Table 5–1 and results in the nonworkers having a higher mortality rate than the remainder of the general population that comprises current workers. In this hypothetical example, workers in the general population have the same mortality rate as the exposed workers at the study plant, but because the nonworkers in the general population have a rate that is five times as great as that of workers, the overall rate in the general population is considerably greater than that of the exposed workers. Thus, in a study that compared the mortality rate of the ex-

Table 5–1. The healthy worker effect is an example of a selection bias that underestimates the mortality related to occupational exposures, as illustrated by these hypothetical rates among workers and the general population

	Exposed Workers	General Population		
		Workers	Nonworkers	Total
Deaths	50	4500	2500	7000
Person-time	1000	90,000	10,000	100,000
Mortality rate (cases/year)	0.05	0.05	0.25	0.07

posed workers with that of the general population, the exposed workers would have a lower mortality rate as a result of this selection bias.

Information Bias

Systematic error in a study can arise because the information collected about or from study subjects is erroneous. Such information is often referred to as being *misclassified* if the variable is measured on a categorical scale and the error leads to a person being placed in an incorrect category. For example, a heavy smoker who is categorized as a light smoker is misclassified. Typically, the two primary variables in an epidemiologic study relate to exposure and disease. Misclassification of subjects for either exposure or disease can be *differential* or *nondifferential.* These terms refer to the mechanism for misclassification. For exposure misclassification, the misclassification is nondifferential if it is unrelated to the occurrence or presence of disease; if the misclassification of exposure is different for those with and without disease, it is differential. Similarly, misclassification of disease is nondifferential if it is unrelated to exposure; otherwise, it is differential.

A common type of information bias is *recall bias,* which occurs in case-control studies where a subject is interviewed to obtain exposure information after disease has occurred. For example, case-control studies of babies born with birth defects sometimes obtain interview information from mothers after the birth. Mothers who have given birth to a baby with a serious birth defect are thought to be able to recall accurately many exposures during early pregnancy, such as taking nonprescription drugs or experiencing a fever, because the adverse pregnancy outcome serves as a stimulus for the mother to consider potential causes. Mothers of normal babies, however, have had no comparable stimulus to search their memories and may consequently fail to recall exposures such as nonprescription drugs or fevers. The discrepancy in recall gives rise to a particular version of recall bias known as *maternal recall bias.* This problem is distinct from the more general problem of remembering and reporting exposures, which affects all people to some extent and tends to be a non-differential, rather than a differential, misclassification.

How can recall bias be prevented? One approach is to frame the questions to aid accurate recall. Improving accuracy of recall will reduce recall bias because it will limit the inaccurate recall among controls. Another approach is to take an entirely different control group that will not be subject to the incomplete recall. For example, mothers of babies born with birth defects other than the one under study may provide recall of earlier exposures comparable with that of case mothers. Yet another approach to avoiding recall bias is to conduct a study that does not use interview information but, instead, information from medical records that was recorded before the birth outcome was known.

Recall bias is a differential misclassification because the exposure information is misclassified differentially for those with and without disease. An analogous type of differential misclassification is *biased follow-up*, in which unexposed people are underdiagnosed for disease more than exposed people. Suppose an investigator uses a cohort study to assess the effect of tobacco smoking on the occurrence of emphysema. Suppose also that the study will ask about medical diagnoses but will not involve any examinations to check the diagnoses. It may happen that emphysema, a diagnosis that is often missed, is more likely to be diagnosed in smokers than in nonsmokers. Both the smokers themselves and their physicians may be inclined to search more thoroughly for respiratory disease because they are concerned about the effects of smoking. As a result, the diagnosis of emphysema might be missed more frequently among nonsmokers, leading to a differential misclassification of disease. Thus, even if smoking did not lead to emphysema, smokers would appear to have a greater incidence rate of emphysema than nonsmokers because of the greater likelihood that emphysema would not be diagnosed in a nonsmoker. This bias could be avoided by conducting examinations for emphysema as part of the study itself, thereby avoiding the biased follow-up.

The above biases are examples of differential misclassification, when either the exposure is misclassified differentially according to a person's disease status or the disease is misclassified differentially according to a person's exposure status. Differential misclassification can either exaggerate or underestimate an effect. A more pervasive type of misclassification, which affects every epidemiologic study to some extent, is nondifferential misclassification. With nondifferential misclassification, either exposure or disease (or both) is misclassified, but the misclassification does not depend on a person's status for the other variable. For example, suppose that the study hypothesis concerns the relation between consumption of red wine and the development of emphysema. (Assume for this example that consumption of red wine is not related to smoking.) Unlike the situation for smoking, there is little reason to suppose that those who drink more or less red wine will have a greater or a lesser tendency to be diagnosed with emphysema if they have it. As a result, although some people with emphysema will not have it diagnosed, the proportion of people who do not have their emphysema diagnosed would be expected to be the same for those who do and who do not drink red wine. The underdiagnosis represents some misclassification of emphysema, but because the tendency for underdiagnosis is the same for exposed and unexposed people, the misclassification of disease is nondifferential. Similarly, if an exposure is misclassified in a way that does not depend on disease status, the exposure misclassification is nondifferential.

Nondifferential misclassification leads to more predictable biases than does differential misclassification. Nondifferential misclassification of a dichotomous exposure tends to produce estimates of the effect that are diluted, or closer to the null or no-effect value than the actual effect. If there is no effect to begin with, then nondifferential misclassification of the exposure will not bias the effect estimate.

The simplest case to consider is nondifferential misclassification of an exposure measured on a dichotomous scale: exposed versus nonexposed. Suppose that an investigator assesses the relation between eating a high-fat diet and subsequent heart attack in a case-control study. Everyone in the study is classified, according to some arbitrary cut-off value of dietary fat intake, as having either a high-fat diet or not. This classification will not be perfectly accurate because it is nearly impossible to avoid some measurement error. In the case of measuring the fat content of a person's diet, there will be substantial error and some people who do not have a high-fat diet may be classified as having one and vice versa. If these misclassifications are not related to whether a person gets a heart attack, they are nondifferential.

The effect of nondifferential misclassification of a dichotomous exposure is illustrated in Table 5–2. On the left are hypothetical data that presume no misclassification with respect to a high-fat diet. The incidence rate ratio (calculated from the odds ratio) is 5.0, indicating a substantially greater mortality rate among those eating a high-fat diet. The center columns show the result if 20% of those who do not eat a high-fat diet were inaccurately classified as eating a high-fat diet. This level of misclassification is higher than one would ordinarily expect, even for an exposure as difficult to measure as diet, but still involves only a small proportion of the subjects. By moving 20% of those from the *No* column to the *Yes* column, the resulting data give a rate ratio of 2.4, less than half as great as the value with the correct data. In terms of the effect part of the risk ratio, the excess risk ratio of 4.0 ($= 5.0 - 1$) has been reduced to 1.4 ($= 2.4 - 1$), which is to say that about two-thirds of the effect has been obscured. Note that we have transferred both 20% of cases and 20% of controls. Nondifferential misclassification of exposure implies that these percentages of misclassified subjects among cases and controls will be equal. If the proportions of cases and controls that were

Table 5–2. Nondifferential misclassification in a hypothetical case-control study

	Correct Classification		Nondifferential Misclassification			
			20% of No → Yes		20% of No → Yes 20% of Yes → No	
	High-Fat Diet		*High-Fat Diet*		*High-Fat Diet*	
	No	**Yes**	**No**	**Yes**	**No**	**Yes**
Heart attack cases	450	250	360	340	410	290
Controls	900	100	720	280	740	260
Rate ratio	5.0		2.4		2.0	

misclassified differed from one another, that would be differential misclassification.

The third set of columns in Table 5–2 adds further nondifferential misclassification: 20% of cases and controls who ate a high-fat diet are misclassified as not having a high-fat diet. This misclassification is added to the misclassification in the other direction, with the result as shown in the right-hand part of the table. With this additional misclassification, the rate ratio has declined to 2.0, even closer to the null value of 1.0, nullifying three-fourths of the effect seen in the correctly classified data.

Nondifferential misclassification of a dichotomous exposure will always bias an effect, if there is one, toward the null value. If the exposure is not dichotomous, there may be bias toward the null value; but there may also be bias away from the null value, depending on the categories to which individuals are misclassified. In general, nondifferential misclassification between two exposure categories will make the effect estimates for those two categories converge toward one another.[1]

Confounding

Confounding is a central issue for epidemiologic study design. A simple definition of *confounding* would be the confusion, or mixing, of effects: this definition implies that the effect of the exposure is mixed together with the effect of another variable, leading to a bias. Let us illustrate confounding with a classic example: the relation between birth order and the occurrence of Down syndrome. Figure 5–2 shows data on birth order and Down syndrome from the work of Stark and Mantel.[2]

These data show a striking trend in prevalence of Down syndrome with increasing birth order, which we might describe as the effect of birth order on the occurrence of Down syndrome. The effect of birth

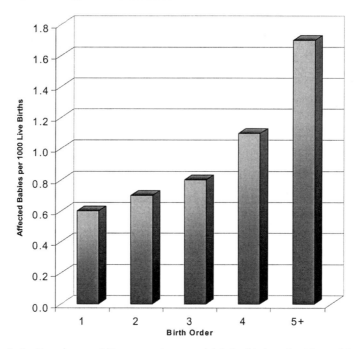

Figure 5–2. Prevalence of Down syndrome at birth by birth order (data of Stark and Mantel[2]).

order, however, is a blend of whatever effect birth order has by itself and the effect of another variable that is closely correlated with birth order. The other variable is the age of the mother. Figure 5–3 gives the relation between mother's age and the occurrence of Down syndrome from the same data. It indicates a much stronger relation between mother's age and Down syndrome: in Figure 5–2, the prevalence increased from about 0.6 per 1000 at the first birth to 1.7 per 1000 for birth order of 5 or greater, a respectably strong trend; in Figure 5–3, however, the prevalence increased from 0.2 per 1000 at the youngest category of mother's age to 8.5 per 1000 at the highest category of mother's age, more than a 40-fold increase. (The vertical scale has changed from Fig. 5–2 to Fig. 5–3.)

Because birth order and the age of the mother are highly correlated, we can expect that mothers giving birth to their fifth baby are, as a group, considerably older than mothers giving birth to their first baby. Therefore, the comparison of high-birth-order babies with lower-birth-order babies is to some extent a comparison of babies born to older mothers with babies born to younger mothers. Thus, the birth-order comparison in Figure 5–2 mixes the effect of mother's age with the effect of birth order. The extent of the mixing depends on the extent to which mother's age is related to birth order. This mixing of effects we call confounding, and we say that the birth-order effect depicted in Figure 5–2 is confounded by the effect of mother's age.

Confounding by indication

Pharmacoepidemiologists study the epidemiology of drug effects, either intended or unintended, often using nonexperimental studies. In such studies, the essential comparisons involve a contrast of outcomes for individuals who have taken a specific drug with those who have not taken the drug. Without a randomized trial, it can be challenging to design a study that yields a valid comparison of drug takers with nontakers. The main challenge comes from a phenomenon that epidemiologists refer to as *confounding by indication*. The problem arises from the fact that those who take a drug generally differ from those who do not according to the medical indication for which the drug was prescribed. Even if the comparison group represents patients with the same disease who received a different therapy or none at all, there will typically be differences in disease severity or other risk factors between populations who receive different treatments. These differences introduce a bias in the comparison that is called confounding by indication.

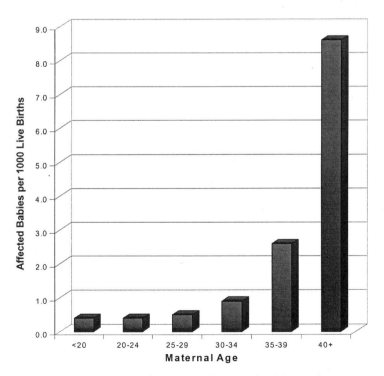

Figure 5–3. Prevalence of Down syndrome at birth by mother's age.

Could we say that the effect of mother's age in Figure 5–3 is also confounded by the effect of birth order? Perhaps. It depends on whether birth order has any effect at all on its own. Because the effect in Figure 5–3 of mother's age is so much stronger than the effect in Figure 5–2 for birth order, we know that birth order cannot fully explain the maternal-age effect, whereas it remains a possibility that maternal age fully accounts for the apparent effect of birth order. A good way to resolve the extent to which one variable's effect explains the apparent effect of the other is to examine both effects simultaneously. Figure 5–4 presents the prevalence of Down syndrome at birth by both birth order and mother's age simultaneously.

Figure 5–4 shows clearly that within each category of birth order, looking from the front to the back, there is the same striking trend in prevalence of Down syndrome with increasing maternal age. In contrast, within each category of maternal age, looking from left to right, there is no discernible trend with birth order. Thus, the apparent trend with birth order in Figure 5–2 was due entirely to confounding by maternal age. On the other hand, there is no confounding in the other direction: birth order does not confound the maternal-age association because birth order has no effect. We call the apparent effect of birth order in Figure 5–2 the *crude effect* of birth order. In Figure 5–4, we can see that within categories of maternal age there is no birth-order effect, so the crude effect in this instance is entirely a result of confounding.

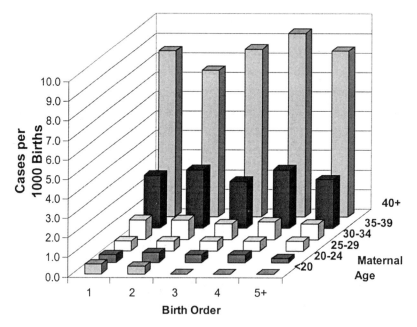

Figure 5–4. Prevalence of Down syndrome at birth by birth order and mother's age.

Is the maternal-age effect in Figure 5–3 confounded? As we have already pointed out, it is not confounded by birth order, which appears to have no effect on its own. On the other hand, it is confounded by other factors. We can be sure of that because age is just a marker of time and time itself does not cause the biologic changes that produce Down syndrome. There must be biologic events that occur during a woman's aging process that lead to the sharp increase in occurrence of Down syndrome among the offspring of older mothers. Mother's age is thus a proxy for as yet unidentified events that more directly account for the occurrence of Down syndrome. When these events are identified, we would ultimately find that mother's age has no effect once we take into account the biologic changes that are correlated with age, which is to say that the apparent effect of mother's age is also confounded by factors as yet unknown.

The research process of learning about and controlling for confounding can be thought of as a walk through a maze toward a central goal. The path through the maze eventually permits the scientist to penetrate into levels that successively get closer to the goal: in this example, the apparent relation between Down syndrome and birth order can be explained entirely by the effect of mother's age, but that effect in turn ultimately will be explained by other factors that have not yet been identified. As the layers of confounding are left behind, we gradually approach a deeper causal understanding of the underlying biology. Unlike a maze, however, this journey toward biologic understanding does not have a clear end point, in the sense that there is always room to understand the biology in a deeper way.

Above, we defined confounding as the confusion, or mixing, of effects. Strictly speaking, the exposure variable may or may not have an effect; in the Down syndrome example, birth order did not have an effect. The confounding variable, however, must have an effect on the outcome to be confounding. Theoretically, a confounding variable should actually be a cause of the disease, but in practice it may be only a proxy or a marker for a cause. That is precisely the case for mother's age, which by itself does not cause Down syndrome but serves as a marker for unknown biologic events that accumulate with time. Whether a cause or a marker for a cause, a confounder will be a predictor of disease occurrence.

Not every predictor of disease occurrence is a confounding factor. For confounding to occur, a predictor of disease occurrence must also be imbalanced across exposure categories. Suppose that age is a risk factor for a given disease (as it usually is). Age would nevertheless not be confounding unless the age distributions of people in the various exposure categories differed. If every exposure category contains people whose age distribution is the same as that for people in other exposure categories, the comparison of disease rates across exposure categories would not be influenced by the age effect. On the other hand, if age is imbalanced across exposure categories, then comparison of one exposure category with another involves people whose age distributions differ. Under those circumstances, the effect of exposure will be confounded with the effect of age to an extent that depends on the strength of the relation between age and the disease as well as the extent of the age imbalance across exposure categories.

Let us consider another example. In 1970, the University Group Diabetes Program published the results of a randomized trial designed to assess how well three treatments for diabetes prevented fatal complications.[3] Table 5–3 presents the crude data comparing one of the treatments, the drug tolbutamide, with placebo, with respect to total mortality over a period that averaged 7 years. The proportion of subjects who died was greater in the tolbutamide group than in the placebo group, a surprising result that spurred a long and bitter controversy and brought tremendous scrutiny to these study results. If we measure the effect of treatment as the difference in the proportion of those who died in the tolbutamide and placebo groups, we estimate an adverse effect of tolbutamide of $0.147 - 0.102 = 0.045$. In other words, this result translates to an estimate that subjects who receive tolbutamide face an additional risk of 4.5% of dying over 7 years compared with subjects who receive placebo.

Although this was a randomized experiment, as it happened the random assignment led to imbalances between the tolbutamide and placebo groups with respect to age. Randomization is intended to balance out potential confounding factors between the compared groups, but it cannot guarantee such a balance. In this case, the tolbutamide group comprised subjects who were older on average than the placebo group. Because age is strongly related to the risk of death, this imbalance in age introduced confounding. In the Down syndrome example above, we were able to remove the confounding by examining the effect of birth order within categories of mother's age. This process is called *stratification*. We can also stratify the data from the University Group Diabetes Program by age (Table 5–4).

From Table 5–4, we can see that of the 204 subjects who received

Table 5–3. Deaths among subjects who received tolbutamide and placebo in the University Group Diabetes Program (1970)

	Tolbutamide	Placebo
Deaths	30	21
Surviving	174	184
Total	204	205
Mortality proportion	0.147	0.102

Table 5–4. Deaths among subjects who received tolbutamide and placebo in the University Group Diabetes Program (1970), stratifying by age

	Age <55 years		Age ≥ 55 years	
	Tolbutamide	**Placebo**	**Tolbutamide**	**Placebo**
Dead	8	5	22	16
Surviving	98	115	76	69
Total	106	120	98	85
Mortality proportion	0.076	0.042	0.224	0.188
Difference in proportion	0.034		0.036	

tolbutamide in the study, 98 (48%), were age 55 or above; in contrast, only 85/205 placebo subjects (41%), were age 55 or above. This difference may not appear striking, but the difference in the risk of dying during the 7 years is strikingly greater for those age 55 or above than for younger subjects. With age so strongly related to the risk of death, the difference in the age distribution is potentially worrisome. Did it lead to confounding by age? To answer that, we can look at the difference in the proportion who died, comparing tolbutamide with placebo, in each of the two age groups. In both groups, there is an approximately 3.5% greater risk of death over the 7 years for the tolbutamide group than for the placebo group. (Actually, the data show a difference of 3.4 % for the younger group and 3.6% for the older group. As a summary measure, we might average these two values and call the overall difference 3.5%. Technically, we would want to take an average that weighted each of the age categories according to the amount of data in that category.) When we ignored age, we found a difference of 4.5%. The value of 4.5% that we obtained from the crude data is confounded and gives an overestimate of the adverse effect of tolbutamide. The value of 3.5% obtained after the age stratification may not be completely unconfounded by age. Because we used only two age categories, it is possible that age differences remain within the age categories in table 5–4. Nevertheless, even with this simple age stratification, the estimate of effect is lower than the estimate from the crude data. The crude data overestimate the adverse effect of tolbutamide by nearly 30% (4.5% is nearly 30% greater than 3.5%). We will return to the topic of stratification in Chapter 8.

The University Group Diabetes Program study illustrates that even randomization cannot prevent confounding in all instances. In this case, it led to an age imbalance, which caused a moderate amount of confounding. The confounding in the Down syndrome example was greater, in large part because the association between mother's age and birth order was stronger than the association between age and tolbutamide that the randomization produced.

Confounding can cause a bias in either direction: it can cause an over-

---

Properties of a confounding factor

Confounding can be thought of as a mixing of effects. A confounding factor, therefore, must have an effect and must be imbalanced between the exposure groups to be compared. In essence, these conditions imply that a confounding factor must have two associations:

- A confounder must be associated with the disease (either as a cause or as a proxy for a cause but not as an effect of the disease).
- A confounder must be associated with the exposure.

There is also a third requirement. A factor that is an effect of the exposure and an intermediate step in the causal pathway from exposure to disease will have the above properties, but causal intermediates are not confounders; they are part of the effect that we wish to study. For example, if a diet high in saturated fat leads to higher levels of low-density lipoprotein (LDL) in the blood and high LDL leads to atherosclerosis, high LDL will be associated with both diet and atherosclerosis. Nevertheless, high LDL does not confound the relation between diet and atherosclerosis; it is part of the exposure's effect and should not be considered confounding. In fact, any effect of the exposure, whether it is part of the causal pathway to the disease or not, is not a confounder. Thus, the third property of a confounder is as follows:

- A confounder must not be an effect of the exposure.

---

estimate of the effect, as the confounder mother's age did for birth order and Down syndrome and the confounder age did for tolbutamide and death; or it can cause an underestimate of the effect, as the confounder age did for smoking and death in the example in Chapter 1. The bias introduced by confounding can, on occasion, be strong enough to reverse the apparent direction of an effect.[4]

Control of Confounding

Confounding is a systematic error that investigators aim either to prevent or to remove from a study. There are two common methods to prevent confounding. One of them, *randomization,* or the random assignment of subjects to experimental groups, can only be used in experiments. The other, *restriction,* involves selecting subjects for a study who have the same value, or nearly the same value, for a variable that might be a confounder. Restriction can be used in any epidemiologic study, regardless of whether it is an experiment or not. (A third method to prevent confounding, *matching,* is an advanced topic that we will not deal with here. One of the reasons that matching is an advanced topic is that, although it does prevent confounding in cohort studies, in case-control studies, surprisingly, it does not. In fact, it can even introduce confounding into case-control studies when there was none to begin with. A thorough discussion of matching can be found in *Modern Epidemiology.*[1])

In experiments where the investigator assigns the exposure to study subjects, randomization confers powerful benefits. With a sufficiently large study population, randomization produces two or more study groups with nearly the same distribution of characteristics. This similarity for all variables implies that the compared groups will be similar for risk factors that predict the outcome of interest and, therefore, that these risk predictors will not confound. Randomization cannot guarantee the absence of confounding: a random process can still lead to confounding imbalances, such as the age imbalance that occurred in the experiment in Table 5–4. The likelihood of a large imbalance, however, becomes small as the number of subjects who are randomized increases. Perhaps the most important benefit of randomization is that it prevents confounding for unidentified factors as well as for factors that are already of concern. Even unknown risk factors will not confound in a randomized experiment of sufficient size.

Restriction, unlike randomization, cannot control for unknown confounding factors. On the other hand, it is more certain to prevent confounding by those factors for which it is employed. For example, in a study of alcohol drinking and cancer of the throat, smoking might be considered a likely confounding variable: smoking is a cause of throat cancer, and people who drink alcohol smoke more than people who do not drink alcohol. If the study were confined to nonsmokers, then smoking could not be a confounder. Similarly, if age is thought to be a likely confounding factor in a study, confounding by age can be prevented by enrolling subjects who are nearly the same age. If everyone in a study has the same value for a variable, then that factor can no longer vary in the study setting; it becomes a constant. For confounding to occur, a confounding factor must be associated with exposure, but if a factor is constant, it will not be associated with anything. Thus, restriction is an effective way to prevent confounding in any study.

Restriction is even used in experiments in addition to randomization, to be certain that confounding for certain factors does not occur. It is also used by laboratory scientists conducting animal experiments, to prevent confounding and enhance the validity of their studies. Typically, a researcher doing an experiment with mice will seek only mice bred from the same lab which have the same genotype, the same age, and sometimes the same sex.

It may appear puzzling that restriction is not used more often in epidemiologic research. One explanation is that many researchers have been taught that an epidemiologic study, whether it be an experiment or a nonexperimental study, should comprise study subjects whose charac-

Is confounding in a randomized experiment a bias?

Earlier in this chapter, we proposed that if an error in a study would decrease if the study were larger, that error is a random error, whereas an error that did not decrease if the study were larger is a systematic error. Confounding is usually considered a systematic error, but confounding in an experiment is an exception. In all types of epidemiologic study, confounding arises from imbalances in risk factors for the outcome across the exposure categories. Uniquely in randomized experiments, however, these imbalances are determined by random assignment. As a result of the law of large numbers, the larger the experiment, the more closely the randomly assigned groups will resemble one another in their distributions of risk factors. Because the amount of confounding depends on the size of the experiment, confounding in an experiment is an example of random error rather than systematic error. For systematic errors, replicating the study replicates the error, but for confounding in an experiment, replicating the study (with a new random assignment) will not replicate the same confounding since there will be an entirely new set of assignments to the study groups. Despite being an example of random error rather than systematic error, confounding in an experiment can be controlled using the same methods to control confounding in nonexperimental studies.

For clarification, in this discussion, a large experiment does not necessarily mean one with many participants but, more specifically, one that has a large number of random assignments. For example, a study may involve the random assignment of a community intervention to eight cities that contain millions of people. With only eight random assignments, however, it is not large enough to prevent substantial confounding.

teristics are representative of the target population for whom the study results are intended. The goal of *representativeness* appears to work contrary to the method of restriction, which would provide a study population that is homogeneous and therefore not similar to most target populations of interest. Representativeness is a fallacy that has plagued epidemiologic studies for decades. As explained in Chapter 2, the notion that representativeness is a worthwhile goal presumably stems from the arena of survey research, in which a sample of a larger population is surveyed to avoid the expense and trouble of surveying the entire population. The statistical inference that such sampling allows is only superficially similar to the scientific inference that is the goal of epidemiologic research. For scientific inference, the goal is not to infer a conclusion that would apply to a specific target population but rather to infer an abstract theory that is not tied to a specific population. One can make a scientific inference more readily without confounding; thus, restriction enhances the ability to make a scientific inference, as those who work with laboratory animals know.

What of the concern that restriction makes it difficult to know whether a studied relation applies to people with characteristics different from those in a study population? For example, suppose that an investigator uses restriction to study the effect of drinking wine on cardiovascular disease risk among people who are 60 years of age. Would the study results apply to people who are 45 years of age? The answer is maybe; without outside knowledge, it might not be possible to say whether the study results apply to people who are 45 years of age. This uncertainty leaves open the possibility of an erroneous or incomplete conclusion, but such is the nature of science. It is nevertheless wrong to think that the theorization needed to apply the results of a study to people with different characteristics could be replaced by mechanical sampling. If one suspects that the effect of wine consumption on cardiovascular risk is different for 60-year-olds and 45-year-olds, one would want to select a group of 45-year-olds to study in addition to the 60-year-olds. The number of study subjects and their age distribution should not reflect the age distribution in some target population: why let the demographics of a locale dictate the age distribution of subjects that one chooses for study? Instead, the investigator can choose to study subjects of whatever age seems interesting and in numbers that suit the study design rather than reflect the numbers of people in a target population at those ages. Scientifically, there is no specific target population. There is instead a scientific theory about wine, cardiovascular disease risk, and perhaps age. It is the theory that is the real target of inference. A valid study is the best route to a correct inference, and restriction, rather than representativeness, is the more desirable means to achieve the correct inference.

If confounding is not controlled adequately in the study design, it may still be possible to control it in the data analysis. To do so requires that the study data include adequate information about the confounding factor(s). Two methods can be used to deal with confounding in the data analysis: one is stratification, a technique illustrated above in Table 5–4 and discussed in Chapter 1 and in greater detail in Chapter 8; the other is to use regression models, an analytic technique that is described in Chapter 10.

Questions

1. Suppose a case-control study could be expanded to be infinitely large. Which sources of error would be eliminated by such a study and which would not? Suppose that a randomized trial could be infinitely large. Which sources of error would remain in such a trial?
2. Will a larger study have less bias than a smaller study? Why or why not?

3. When recall bias occurs, patients who have been afflicted with a medical problem, such as a heart attack, give responses about possible causes of that problem that differ from those given by nonafflicted subjects. Whose responses are thought to be more accurate?
4. Suppose that in analyzing the data from an epidemiologic study, a computer coding error led to the exposed group being classified as unexposed and the unexposed group being classified as exposed. What effect would this error have on the reported results (be specific)? Is this a bias? If so, what type; if not, what type of error is it?
5. Explain the difference between a confounding factor and a potential confounding factor. In what situations might a potential confounding factor not end up being a confounding factor?
6. The incidence rate of cardiovascular disease increases with increasing age. Does that mean that age will always confound studies of cardiovascular disease in the same direction? Why or why not?
7. The effectiveness of randomization in controlling confounding depends on the size of the experiment. Consider an experiment to study the impact of nutritional education of schoolchildren on their serum cholesterol levels. Suppose that the study involved randomly assigning 10 classrooms with 30 children each to receive a new curriculum and another 10 classrooms with 30 children each to receive the old curriculum. Should this be considered a study that compares two groups with 300 in each group or 10 in each group, from the viewpoint of the effectiveness of controlling confounding by randomization?
8. Confounding by indication arises because those who take a given drug differ for medical reasons from those who do not take the drug. Is this problem truly confounding, or is it more appropriately described as a selection bias?
9. Those who favor representative studies claim that one cannot generalize a study to a population whose characteristics differ from those of the study population. Thus, a study of smoking and lung cancer in men would tell nothing about the relation between smoking and lung cancer in women. Give the counterarguments. (Hint: If the study were conducted in London, would the results apply to those who lived in Paris?)

References

1. Rothman, KJ, Greenland, S: *Modern Epidemiology, 2nd ed.* Philadelphia: Lippincott, 1998.
2. Stark, CR, Mantel, N: Effects of maternal age and birth order on the risk of mongolism and leukemia. *J Natl Cancer Inst* 1966;37:687–698.
3. University Group Diabetes Program. A study of the effects of hypoglycemic agents on vascular complications in patients with adult onset diabetes. *Diabetes* 1970;19(Suppl. 2):747–830.
4. Reintjes, R, de Boer, A, van Pelt, W, et al: Simpson's paradox: an example from hospital epidemiology. *Epidemiology* 2000;11:81–83.

6

Random Error and the Role
of Statistics

Statistics plays two main roles in the analysis of epidemiologic data: one is to assess variability in the data, in an effort to distinguish chance findings from results that might be replicated upon repetition of the work; the other is to estimate effects after correcting for biases such as confounding. In this chapter, we concentrate on the assessment of variability. The use of statistical approaches to control confounding will be discussed in Chapters 8 and 10.

An epidemiologic study can be viewed as an exercise in measurement, as we saw in the preceding chapters. As in any measurement, the goal is to obtain an accurate result, with as little error as possible. Both systematic error and random error can distort the measurement process. Chapter 5 described the primary categories of systematic error. The error that remains after systematic error is eliminated is what we call *random error*. Random error is actually nothing more than variability in the data that we cannot readily explain. Sometimes random error stems from a random process, but it might not. In randomized trials, some of the variability in the data will reflect the random assignment of subjects to the study groups. In most epidemiologic studies, however, there is no random assignment to study groups. For example, in a cohort study that compares the outcome of pregnancy among women who drink heavily chlorinated water with the outcome among women who drink bottled water, it is not chance but the decision-making or circumstances of the women themselves that determines the cohort into which the women fall. The individual "assignments" to categories of water chlorination are not random; nevertheless, we still consider some of the variability in the outcome to be random error. Much of this variation may reflect hidden biases and presumably can be accounted for by factors other than drinking water that affect the outcome of pregnancy. These factors may not have been measured among these women, or perhaps not even discovered.

Estimation

If an epidemiologic study is thought of as an exercise in measurement, then the result should provide an estimate of an epidemiologic quantity. Ideally, the analysis of data and the reporting of results should quantify the magnitude of that epidemiologic quantity and portray the degree of precision with which it is measured. Estimation provides these quantities. For example, a case-control study might be undertaken to estimate the incidence rate ratio (RR) between use of cellular telephones and the occurrence of brain cancer. The report on the results of the study should present a clear estimate of the RR, such as RR = 2.5. When an estimate is presented as a single value, we refer to it as a *point estimate*. In this example, the point estimate of 2.5 quantifies the estimated strength of the relation between the use of cellular telephones and the occurrence of brain cancer. To indicate the precision of the point estimate, we use a *confidence interval*, which is a range of values around the point estimate. A wide confidence interval indicates low precision, and a narrow interval indicates high precision.

Point Estimates, Confidence Intervals, and p Values

The reason that we need confidence intervals is that a point estimate, being a single value, cannot express the statistical variation, or random error, that underlies the estimate. If a study is large, the estimation process would be comparatively precise and there would be little random error in the estimation. A small study, however, would have less precision, which is to say that the estimate would be subject to more random error. We use a confidence interval to indicate the amount of random error in the estimate. A given confidence interval is tied to an arbitrarily set level of confidence. Commonly, the arbitrary level of confidence is set at either 95% or 90%, although any level in the interval 0%–100% is possible. The confidence interval is defined statistically as follows: if the level of confidence is set at 95%, it means that if the data collection and analysis could be replicated many times, the confidence interval should include within it the correct value of the measure 95% of the time. This definition presumes that the only thing that would differ in these hypothetical replications of the study would be the statistical, or chance, element in the data. It also presumes that the variability in the data can be described adequately by a statistical model and that biases such as confounding are nonexistent. These unrealistic conditions are typically not met even in carefully designed and conducted randomized trials. In nonexperimental epidemiologic studies, the formal definition of a confidence interval is a fiction that at best provides a rough estimate of the statistical variability in a set of data. It is better not to consider a confi-

---

Chance

In ordinary language, the word *chance* has a dual meaning: one refers to the outcome of a random process, implying an outcome that could not be predicted under any circumstances; the other refers to outcomes that cannot be predicted easily but are not necessarily random phenomena. For example, if you unexpectedly encounter your cousin on the beach at Cape Cod, you may describe it as a chance encounter. Nevertheless, there were presumably causal mechanisms that can explain why both you and your cousin were on the beach at Cape Cod at that time. It may be a coincidence that the two causal mechanisms led to your both being there together, but randomness does not necessarily play a role in explaining the encounter.

We might consider the flip of a coin to be a randomizing event, one that is completely unpredictable. In fact, however, the flip of a coin can be predicted with sufficient information about the initial conditions and the forces applied to the coin. Indeed, some individuals have practiced flipping coins enough to predict the outcome nearly perfectly. For most of us, the flip of a coin seems random, despite the fact that the process is not. As we practice flipping or learn more about the sources of error in a body of data, we can reduce the apparently random error. Physicists tell us that we will never be able to explain all components of error, but for the problems that epidemiologists address, it is reasonable to assume that much of the random error that we observe in data could be explained with better information.

---

dence interval to be a literal measure of statistical variability but rather a general guide to the amount of error in the data.

The confidence interval is calculated from the same equations used to generate another commonly reported statistical measure, the *p value,* which is the statistic used for hypothesis testing. The *p* value is calculated in relation to a specific hypothesis, usually the *null hypothesis,* which states that there is no relation between exposure and disease. For the RR measure, the null hypothesis is RR $= 1.0$. The *p* value represents the probability, assuming that the null hypothesis is true, that the data obtained in a study would demonstrate an association as far from the null hypothesis as, or farther than, what was actually obtained. For example, suppose that a case-control study gives 2.5 as an estimate of the relative risk. The *p* value answers the question "What is the probability, if the relative risk is 1.0, that a study might give a result as far as this, or farther, from 1.0?" Thus, the *p* value is the probability, conditional on the null hypothesis, of observing as strong an association as was observed or a stronger one.

We calculate p values using statistical models that correspond to the type of data collected (see Chapter 7). In practice, the variability of collected data is unlikely to conform precisely to any given statistical model. For example, most statistical models assume that the observations are independent of one another. Many epidemiologic studies, however, are based on observations that are not independent. In addition, the data could be influenced by systematic errors that increase variation beyond that expected from a simple statistical model. Thus, because the theoretical requirements are seldom met, a p value usually cannot be taken as a meaningful probability value. Instead, it could be viewed as something less technical: a measure of relative consistency between the null hypothesis and the data in hand. Thus, a large p value indicates that the data are highly consistent with the null hypothesis, and a low p value indicates that the data are not very consistent with the null hypothesis. More specifically, if a p value were as small as 0.01, it would mean that the data are not very consistent with the null hypothesis, but a p value as large as 0.5 would indicate that the data are reasonably consistent with the null hypothesis. Neither of these p values ought to be interpreted as a strict probability. Neither tells us whether the null hypothesis is correct or not. The ultimate judgment about the correctness of the null hypothesis will depend on the existence of other data and the relative plausibility of the null hypothesis and its alternatives.

Statistical Hypothesis Testing versus Estimation

Often, a p value is used to determine the presence or absence of *statistical significance*. *Statistical significance* is a term that appears laden with meaning but, in fact, tells nothing more than whether the p value is less than some arbitrary value, almost always 0.05. Thus, the term *statistically significant* and the statement $p < 0.05$ (or whatever level is taken as the threshold for statistical significance) are equivalent. Neither is a good description of the information in the data.

Statistical hypothesis testing is a term used to describe the process of deciding whether to reject or not to reject a specific hypothesis, usually the null hypothesis. Statistical hypothesis testing is predicated on statistical significance as determined from the p value. Typically, if an analysis gives a result that is statistically significant, the null hypothesis is rejected as false. If a result is not statistically significant, it means that the null hypothesis cannot be rejected. It does not mean that the null hypothesis is correct. No data analysis can determine definitively whether the null hypothesis, or any hypothesis, is true or false. Nevertheless, it is unfortunately often the case that a statistical significance test is interpreted to mean that the null hypothesis is either false or true, according to whether the statistical test of the relation between exposure and disease is or is not statistically significant. In practice, a statistical test, ac-

What is the probability that the null hypothesis is correct?

Here is a statement paraphrasing what a public-health official said about a study showing the risks of birth defects among babies born to mothers drinking polluted water: "There is only a 1% probability that the association in this study was produced by chance." The official was referring to the fact that the p value in the study was 0.01. The official's statement is equivalent to saying that there is only a 1% probability that the null hypothesis is correct, and it implies that the p value is equivalent to the probability that the null hypothesis is correct. Unfortunately, that is not so.

True, the p value is supposed to be a probability measure. Furthermore, when the data are very discrepant with the null hypothesis, the p value is small, and when the data are concordant with the null hypothesis, the p value is large. Nonetheless, the p value is not the probability that the null hypothesis is correct. The p value is calculated only after assuming that the null hypothesis is correct; it refers to the probability that data could deviate from the null hypothesis as much as they did or more. It can thus be viewed as a measure of consistency between the data and the null hypothesis. It does not describe the probability that the null hypothesis is correct, however. The null hypothesis may be the most reasonable hypothesis for the data even if the p value is low, or it may be implausible or just incorrect even if the p value is high.

companied by its declaration of "significant" or "not significant," is often mistakenly used as a forced decision on the truth of the null hypothesis.

A declaration of statistical significance offers less information than the p value because the p value is a number, whereas statistical significance is just a dichotomous description. There is no reason that the numerical p value must be degraded into this less informative dichotomy. Even the more quantitative p value has a problem, however: it confounds two important aspects of the data, the strength of the relation between exposure and disease and the precision with which that relation is measured. To have a clear interpretation of data, it is important to be able to separate the information on strength of relation and precision, which is the job that estimation does for us.

p Value (Confidence Interval) Functions

To illustrate how estimation does a better job of expressing both strength of relation and precision, we will describe a curve that is often called a p *value function* but is also referred to as a *confidence interval function*. It will become clear why this curve merits both names. The p value function enlarges upon the concept of the p value. As stated above, the p value is a statistic that can be viewed as a measure of the compatibility between the data in hand and the null hypothesis. We can enlarge upon this concept by imagining that instead of testing just the null hypothesis, we calculate a p value for a range of other hypotheses as well. Suppose we consider the rate ratio measure, which can range from 0 to infinity and equals 1.0 if the null hypothesis is correct. The ordinary p value is a measure of the consistency between the data and the hypothesis that RR = 1.0. Mathematically, however, we are not constrained to test only the hypothesis that RR = 1.0. For any set of data, we could, in principle, calculate a p value that measures the compatibility between those data and any value of RR. Not only could we test any particular value of RR, we could, in fact, calculate an infinite number of p values that test every possible value of RR. If we did so and plotted the results, we would end up with the p value function. An example of a p value function is given in Figure 6–1, which is based on the data in Table 6–1 describing a case-control study of drug exposure during pregnancy and congenital heart disease.[1]

The curve in Figure 6–1 plots the p value testing the compatibility of the data in Table 6–1 with every possible value of RR. Where RR = 1.0, the curve gives the p value testing the hypothesis that RR = 1.0; this is the usual p value, testing the null hypothesis. The curve, which resembles a tepee, also gives the p values testing every possible value of RR. Note that for the data depicted in Figure 6–1, the ordinary p value is 0.08. This value would be described by many observers as "not significant" because it is greater than 0.05. To many people, "not significant" implies that there is no relation between exposure and disease in the data. It is a fallacy, however, to infer a lack of association from a p value. In fact, the full p value function in Figure 6–1 makes it clear that there is a strong association in the data, despite the p value being greater than 0.05. The curve gives the p value that would result from testing the compatibility between the data and every possible value of RR. Where the curve reaches its maximum (for which p = 1.0), we have the value of the RR that is most compatible with the observed data. This RR value is called the point estimate. In the figure, we can see that the point estimate is RR = 3.2. As the RR departs from the point estimate in either direction, the p values decline, indicating less compatibility between the data and these RR hypotheses. The curve provides a quantitative overview of the statistical relation between exposure and disease. It indicates the best single value for RR based on the data, and it gives a visual appreciation of the degree of precision of the estimate, which is indicated by the narrowness or broadness of the tepee.

The curve in Figure 6–1 indicates that the p value testing the hypothesis that RR = 1.0 is 0.08. Those who rely on statistical significance for their interpretation of data might take this "nonsignificant" p value to

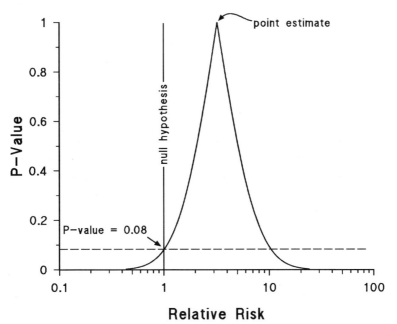

Figure 6–1. *p* value function for the case-control data in Table 6–1.

mean that there is no relation between exposure and disease. That interpretation is already contradicted by the point estimate, which indicates
that the best estimate is more than a threefold increase in risk among
those who are exposed. Moreover, the *p* value function shows that RR
values that are reasonably compatible with the data extend over a wide
range, roughly from RR = 1 to RR = 10. Indeed, the *p* value for RR =
1 is identical to that for RR = 10.5, so there is no reason to prefer the
interpretation RR = 1 over the interpretation RR = 10.5. Of course, a
better estimate than either of these is RR = 3.2, the point estimate. The

Table 6–1. Case-control data from a study on
congenital heart disease and chlordiazopoxide
use in early pregnancy*

| | Chlordiazopoxide Use | | |
	Yes	No	Total
Cases	4	386	390
Controls	4	1250	1254
Total	8	1636	1644

OR = (4 × 1250) / (4 × 386) = 3.2

*Data from Rothman et al.[2]

main lesson here is how misleading it can be to base an inference on a test of statistical significance or, for that matter, on a *p* value.

This lesson is reinforced when we consider another *p* value function that describes a set of hypothetical data, given in Table 6–2. These hypothetical data lead to a narrow *p* value function that reaches a peak slightly above the null value, RR = 1. Figure 6–2 contrasts the *p* value function for the data in Table 6–2 with that given earlier for the data in Table 6–1. The narrowness of the second *p* value function reflects the larger size of the second set of data. Large size translates into better precision, for which the visual counterpart is the narrow *p* value function.

There is a striking contrast in messages from these two *p* value functions. The first function suggests that the data are imprecise but reflect an association that is strong; the data are readily compatible with a wide range of effects, from very little or nothing to more than a 10-fold increase in risk. The first set of data thus raises the possibility that the exposure is a strong risk factor. Although the data do not permit a precise estimate of effect, the range of effect values consistent with the data includes mostly strong effects that would warrant concern about the exposure. This concern comes from data that give a "nonsignificant" result for a test of the null hypothesis. In contrast, the other set of data, from Table 6–2, gives a precise estimate of an effect that is close to the null. The data are not very compatible with a strong effect and, indeed, may be interpreted as reassuring about the absence of a strong effect. Despite this reassurance, the *p* value testing the null hypothesis is 0.04; thus, a test of the null hypothesis would give a "statistically significant" result, rejecting the null hypothesis. In both of these cases, reliance on the significance test would be misleading and conducive to an incorrect interpretation. In the first case, the association is "not significant," but the study is properly interpreted as raising concern about the effect of the exposure. In the second case, the study actually provides reassurance about the absence of a strong effect, but the significance test gives a result that is "significant," rejecting the null hypothesis. This perverse behavior of the significance test should serve as a warning against using significance tests to interpret data.

Table 6–2. Hypothetical case-control data

	Exposed	Unexposed	Total
Cases	1090	14,910	16,000
Controls	1000	15,000	16,000
Total	2090	29,910	32,000

OR = (1090 × 15,000) / (1000 × 14,910) = 1.1

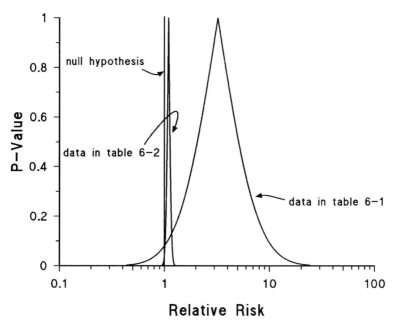

Figure 6–2. *p* value function for the data in Table 6–1 and the hypothetical case-control data in Table 6–2.

Although it may superficially seem like a sophisticated application of quantitative methods, significance testing is only a qualitative proposition. The end result is a declaration of "significant" or "not significant" that provides no quantitative clue about the size of the effect. Contrast that approach with the most quantitative estimate that we can provide: the *p* value function. It presents a quantitative visual message about the estimated size of the effect. The message comes in two parts, relating to the strength of the effect and the precision. Strength is conveyed by the location of the curve along the horizontal axis and precision by the spread of the function around the point estimate. Because the *p* value is only one number, it cannot convey two separate quantitative messages.

To get the message about both strength of effect and precision, at least two numbers are required. Perhaps the most straightforward way to get both messages is from the two numbers that form the boundaries to a confidence interval. The *p* value function is closely related to the set of all confidence intervals for a given estimate. This relation is depicted in Figure 6–3, which shows three different confidence intervals for the data in Figure 6–1. These three confidence intervals differ only in the arbitrary level of confidence that determines the width of the interval. In the figure, the 95% confidence interval can be read from the curve along the horizontal line where *p* = 0.05 and the 90% and 80% intervals along the lines where *p* = 0.1 and 0.2, respectively. The different confidence intervals in Figure 6–3 reflect the same degree of precision but differ in

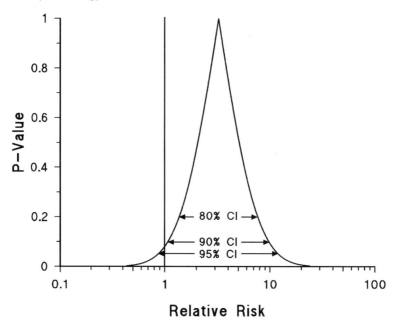

Figure 6–3. *p* value function for the data in Table 6–1, showing how nested confidence intervals can be read from the curve.

their width only in that the level of confidence is arbitrarily different. The three confidence intervals depicted in Figure 6–3 are described as "nested" confidence intervals. The *p* value function can be seen to be a graph of all possible nested confidence intervals for a given estimate, reflecting all possible levels of confidence between 0% and 100%. It is this ability to find all possible confidence intervals from a *p* value function that leads to its description as either a *p* value function or a confidence interval function.

It is common to see confidence intervals reported for an epidemiologic measure, but it is uncommon to see a full *p* value function or confidence interval function. Fortunately, it is not necessary to calculate and display a full *p* value function to infer the two quantitative messages, strength of relation and precision, in an estimate. A single confidence interval is sufficient to do the job, because the upper and lower confidence bounds from a single interval are sufficient to determine the entire *p* value function. If we know the lower and upper limits to the confidence interval, we know both the location of the *p* value function along the horizontal axis and the spread of the function. Thus, from a single confidence interval, we can construct an entire *p* value function. Furthermore, we do not need to go through the labor of constructing this function if we can visualize the two messages that it conveys, both of which can be taken directly from a single confidence interval.

Regrettably, confidence intervals are often not interpreted with the image of a p value function in mind. A confidence interval can unfortunately be used as a surrogate test of statistical significance: a confidence interval that contains the null value within it corresponds to a significance test that is "not significant" and a confidence interval that excludes the null value corresponds to a significance test that is "significant." The allure of significance testing is so strong that many people use a confidence interval merely to determine "significance," and thereby ignore the potentially useful quantitative information that it provides.

Example: Is Flutamide Effective in Treating Prostate Cancer?

In a randomized trial of flutamide, which is used to treat prostate cancer, Eisenberger et al.[2] reported that patients who received flutamide fared no better than those who received placebo. Their interpretation that flutamide was ineffective contradicted the results of 10 previous studies, which had pointed to a modest benefit. The 10 previous studies, on aggregate, indicated about an 11% survival advantage for patients receiving flutamide [odds ratio (OR) = 0.89]). The actual data reported by Eisenberger et al.[2] are given in Table 6–3. From these data, we can calculate an OR of 0.87, nearly the same result (in fact, slightly better) as had been obtained in the 10 earlier studies. (Note: we usually calculate ORs only for case-control data; for these data from an experiment, we normally would calculate either risk ratios or mortality rate ratios. The meta-analysis of the first 10 experiments on flutamide, however, reported only the OR, so we use that measure now for consistency.) Why did Eisenberger et al.[2] interpret their data to indicate no effect when the data indicated about the same beneficial effect as the 10 previous studies? They based their conclusion solely on a test of statistical significance, which gave a result of $p = 0.14$. By focusing on statistical significance testing, they ignored the small beneficial effect in their data and came to an incorrect interpretation.

The original 10 studies on flutamide were published in a review that

Table 6–3. Summary of survival data from a study of flutamide and prostate cancer*

	Flutamide	Placebo
Died	468	480
Survived	229	205
Total	697	685

OR = 0.87
95% CI 0.70–1.10

*Data from Eisenberger et al.[2]

summarized the results.[3] It is helpful to examine the p value function from these 10 studies and to compare it with the p value function after adding the results of Eisenberger et al.[2] to the earlier studies (Figure 6–4).[4] The only change apparent from adding the data of Eisenberger et al.[2] is a slightly improved precision of the estimated benefit of flutamide in reducing the risk of dying from prostate cancer.

Example: Is St. John's Wort Effective at Relieving Major Depression?

Extracts of St. John's wort (*Hypericum perforatum*), a small flowering weed, have long been used as a folk remedy. It is a popular herbal treatment for depression. Shelton and colleagues[5] reported the results of a randomized trial of 200 patients with major depression who were randomly assigned to receive either St. John's wort or placebo. Of 98 who received St. John's wort, 26 responded positively, whereas 19 of the 102 who received placebo responded positively. Among those whose depression was relatively less severe at entry into the study (a group that the

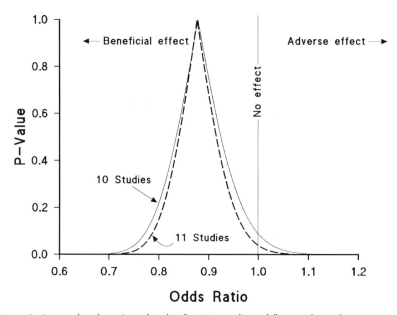

Figure 6–4. p value functions for the first 10 studies of flutamide and prostate cancer survival (*solid line*)[3] and for the first 11 studies having added the data of Eisenberger et al. (*dashed line*).[2] The data of Eisenberger et al. did not shift the overall findings toward the null value but rather shifted the overall findings a minuscule step away from the null. Nevertheless, because of an inappropriate reliance on statistical significance testing, the data were incorrectly interpreted as refuting earlier studies and indicating no effect of flutamide, despite the fact that they replicated previous results.[4] (Reproduced with permission, *The Lancet*, copyright 1999, Elsevier Science, all rights reserved.)

authors thought might be more likely to show an effect of St. John's wort), the proportion who had remission of disease was twice as great among the 59 patients who received St. John's wort as among the 50 who received a placebo (Table 6–4).

In Table 6–4, "risk ratio" refers to the "risk" of having a remission, so any increase above 1.0 indicates a beneficial effect of St. John's wort; the RR of 2.0 indicates that the probability of a remission was twice as great for those receiving St. John's wort. Despite these and other encouraging findings, the authors based their interpretation on a lack of statistical significance and concluded that St. John's wort was not effective. A look at the p value function that corresponds to the data in Table 6–4 is instructive (Figure 6–5).

Figure 6–5 shows that the data regarding remissions among the less severely affected patients hardly support the theory that St. John's wort is ineffective. The data for other outcomes were also generally favorable for St. John's wort but, for nearly all comparisons, not statistically significant. Instead of concluding, as they should have, that these data are readily compatible with moderate and even strong beneficial effects of St. John's wort, the authors drew the wrong conclusion, based on the lack of statistical significance in the data. True, the p value is not statistically significant, but the p value for the null hypothesis is the same as the p value testing the hypothesis that the risk ratio is 4.1. (On the graph, the dashed line intersects the p value function at risk ratios of 1.0 and 4.1.) That is, although the authors interpreted the data as supporting the hypothesis that the risk ratio is 1.0, the data are equally compatible with values of 1.0 and 4.1. Furthermore, it is not necessary to construct the p value function in Figure 6–5 to reach this interpretation. One need look no further than the confidence interval given in Table 6–4 to appreciate the location and spread of the underlying p value function.

Simple Approaches to Calculating Confidence Intervals

In the following chapters, we present basic methods for analyzing epidemiologic data. The focus is on estimating epidemiologic measures of

Table 6–4. Remissions among patients with less severe depression*

	St. John's Wort	Placebo
Remission	12	5
No remission	47	45
Total	59	50

Risk ratio = 2.0
90% CI 0.90–4.6

*Data from Shelton et al.[5]

Statistical significance testing versus estimation

Statistical significance testing is so ingrained that it is nearly ubiqui-tous. Even those who acknowledge the impropriety of basing a conclu-sion on the results of a statistical significance test often fall into the bad habit of equating a lack of significance with a lack of effect and the presence of significance with "proof" of an effect. Significance testing evaluates only one theory that is an alternative to causation to explain the data, the theory that chance accounts for the findings. Nonchance alternative theories, such as confounding, selection bias, and bias from measurement error are all more important to consider. For example, if an investigator finds a "non-significant" result and consequently does not explore it further, he or she may be ignoring an important and even strong association that has been underestimated because of con-founding or nondifferential misclassification. To evaluate these issues, it is crucial to take a quantitative view of the data and their interpreta-tion. That is, it is essential to think in terms of estimation rather than testing.

Significance testing is qualitative, not quantitative. When p values are calculated, they are often reported using inequalities, such as $p < 0.05$, rather than equalities, such as $p = 0.023$. Nothing is gained by converting the continuous p value measure into a dichotomy, but even the numerical p value is far inferior to an estimate of effect, such as that obtained from a confidence interval. Estimation using confi-dence intervals allows one to quantify separately the strength of a rela-tion and the precision of an estimate and, thus, to reach a more reason-able interpretation. The key issue in interpreting a confidence interval is not to take the limits of the interval too literally. Instead of sharp demarcation boundaries, they should be considered gray zones. Ideally, a confidence interval should be viewed as a tool to conjure up an im-age of the full p value function, a smooth curve with no boundary on the estimate. In nearly all instances, there is no need for any test of statistical significance to be calculated, reported, or relied upon, and we are much better off without them.

effect, such as risk and rate ratios and, in cohort studies, risk and rate differences. The overall strategy in a data analysis is to obtain, first, a good point estimate of the epidemiologic measure that we seek and, second, an appropriate confidence interval.

Confidence intervals are usually calculated on the presumption that the estimate comes from the statistical distribution that we call a *normal distribution*, the usual bell-shaped curve. Estimates based on the normal distribution are always reasonable with enough data. When data are sparse, it may be necessary to use more specialized formulas for small

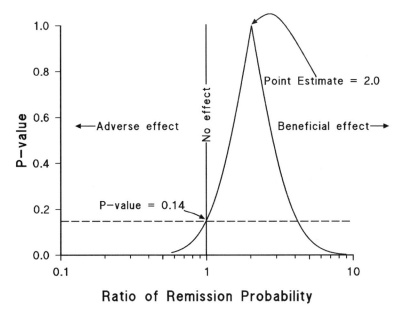

Figure 6–5. *p* value function for the effect of St. John's wort on remission of major depression among relatively less severely affected patients (data of Shelton et al.[5]).

numbers (usually called *exact methods*), but such situations are the exception rather than the rule. A given normal distribution is described with regard to its mean, or center point, and its spread, or *standard deviation* (*standard error* is an equivalent term for *standard deviation* in the applications discussed here).

Suppose that we are estimating the confidence interval for an incidence rate difference, RD. We can use basic formulas to calculate an estimate of the standard deviation (SD) of the RD from the data, and from the SD we can calculate a confidence interval around the point estimate. If we wish to calculate a 95% confidence interval, we would add and subtract 1.96 × SD to the point estimate to get the 95% confidence limits. The value 1.96 is a constant multiplier for the SD that determines an interval encompassing 95% of the normal distribution. If we wish a different level of confidence for the interval, we would use a different multiplier. For example, the multiplier 1.645 corresponds to 90% confidence.

Thus, we would have the following formula for a 90% confidence interval for the rate difference.

$$RD_L, RD_U = RD \pm 1.645 \times SD \qquad (6\text{--}1)$$

In this equation, RD_L refers to the lower confidence limit, obtained using the minus sign, and RD_U refers to the upper confidence limit, obtained using the plus sign. We use the point estimate of RD as the center point for the interval. If 95% confidence limits had been desired, the value 1.96 would be substituted for 1.645. The values for the RD point estimate and for the SD would be calculated from the data, as will be demonstrated in the following chapters.

The above equation is the same general form that would be used to calculate either risk differences or rate differences. We modify this equation slightly, however, when we estimate risk or rate ratios. The reason is that for small or moderate amounts of data the distribution of ratio measures is asymmetrically skewed toward large values. To counteract the skewness, it is customary to set the confidence limits on the log scale, that is, after a logarithmic transformation. Thus, for the RR, we would use the following equation to determine a 90% confidence interval.

$$\ln(RR_L), \ln(RR_U) = \ln(RR) \pm 1.645 \times SD[\ln(RR)]$$

The term $\ln()$ refers to the natural logarithm transformation. A natural logarithm is a logarithm using the base $e \approx 2.7183$. Because this equation will give confidence limits on the log scale, the limits need to be converted back to the RR scale after they are calculated, by reversing the transformation, which involves taking antilogarithms. The whole process can be summarized by the following equation (for a 90% confidence interval):

$$RR_L, RR_U = e^{\ln(RR) \pm 1.645 \times SD[\ln(RR)]} \qquad (6\text{--}2)$$

In the next chapter, we apply these equations to the analysis of simple epidemiologic data.

Questions

1. Why should confidence intervals and p values have a different interpretation in a case-control study or a cohort study than a randomized experiment? What is the impact of the difference on the interpretation?
2. Which has more interpretive value, a confidence interval, a p value, or a statement about statistical significance? Explain.
3. In what way is a p value inherently confounded?
4. What are the two main messages that should come with a statistical estimate? How are these two messages conveyed by a p value function?
5. Suppose that a study showed that former professional football players experienced a rate ratio for coronary heart disease of 3.0 compared with science teachers of the same age and sex, with a 90% confidence interval of 1.0–9.0. Sketch the p value function. What is your interpretation of this finding, presuming that there is no confounding or other obvious bias that distorts the results.
6. One argument sometimes offered in favor of statistical significance testing is that it is often necessary to come to a yes-or-no decision

about the effect of a given exposure or therapy. Significance testing has the apparent benefit of providing a dichotomous interpretation that could be used to make a yes-or-no decision. Comment on the validity of the argument that a decision is sometimes needed based on a research study. What would be the pros and cons of using statistical significance to judge whether an exposure or a therapy has an effect?

7. Are confidence intervals always symmetrical around the point estimate? Why or why not?
8. What is the problem with using a confidence interval to determine whether or not the null value lies within the interval?

References

1. Rothman, KJ, Fyler, DC, Goldblatt, A, et al: Exogenous hormones and other drug exposures of children with congenital heart disease. *Am J Epidemiol* 1979;109:433–439.
2. Eisenberger, MA, Blumenstein, BA, Crawford, ED, et al: Bilateral orchiectomy with or without flutamide for metastatic prostate cancer. *N Engl J Med* 1998;339:1036–1042.
3. Prostate Cancer Trialists' Collaborative Group: Maximum androgen blockade in advanced prostate cancer: an overview of 22 randomised trials with 3283 deaths in 5710 patients. *Lancet* 1995;346:265–269.
4. Rothman, KJ, Johnson, ES, Sugano, DS: Is flutamide effective in patients with bilateral orchiectomy? *Lancet* 1999;353:1184.
5. Shelton, RC, Keller, MB, Gelenberg, A, et al: Effectiveness of St. John's wort in major depression: a randomized controlled trial. *JAMA* 2001;285:1978–1986.

7

Analyzing Simple Epidemiologic Data

In this chapter, we provide the statistical tools to analyze simple epidemiologic data. By simple data, we refer to the most elementary data that could be obtained from an epidemiologic study, such as crude data from a study with no confounding. Because our emphasis is on estimation as opposed to statistical significance testing, we concentrate on formulas for obtaining confidence intervals for basic epidemiologic measures, although we also include formulas to derive p values.

The formulas presented here give only approximate results and are valid only for data with sufficiently large numbers. More accurate estimates can be obtained using what is called *exact* methods. It is difficult to determine a precise threshold of data above which we can say that the approximate results are good enough and below which we can say that exact calculations are needed. Fortunately, even for studies with modest numbers, the interpretation of results rarely changes when exact rather than approximate results are used to estimate confidence intervals. True, for those who place emphasis on whether a confidence interval contains the null value (thereby converting the confidence interval into a statistical test), it may appear to matter if the limit changes its value slightly with a different formula and the limit is near the null value, a situation equivalent to being on the borderline of "statistical significance." As explained in the previous chapter, however, placing emphasis on the exact location of a confidence interval, that is, placing emphasis on statistical significance, is an inappropriate and potentially misleading way to interpret data. With proper interpretation, which ignores the precise location of a confidence limit and instead considers the general width and location of an interval, the difference between results from approximate and exact formulas becomes much less important.

Confidence Intervals for Measures of Disease Frequency

Risk Data (and Prevalence Data)

Suppose we observe that 20 people out of 100 become ill with influenza during the winter season. We would estimate the risk, R, of influenza to be 20/100 or 0.2. To obtain a confidence interval, we need to apply a statistical model. For risk data, the model usually applied is the binomial model. To use the model to obtain a confidence interval, it helps to have some simple notation. Let us use a to represent cases and N to represent people at risk. Using this notation, our estimate of risk would be the number of cases divided by the total number of people at risk: $R = a/N$. We can calculate a confidence interval for the lower and upper confidence limits of R using the following formula.

$$R_L, R_U = R \pm Z \cdot \text{SE}(R) \qquad (7\text{--}1)$$

In this expression, the minus sign is used to obtain the lower confidence limit and the plus sign is used to obtain the upper confidence limit. Z is a fixed value, taken from the standard normal distribution, that determines the confidence level. If Z is set at 1.645, the result is a 90% confidence interval; if it is set at 1.96, the result is a 95% confidence interval. $\text{SE}(R)$ is the *standard error* of R. The standard error is a measure of the statistical variability of estimate. Under the binomial model, the standard error of R would be as follows.

$$\text{SE}(R) = \sqrt{\frac{a(N - a)}{N^3}}$$

Example: Confidence Limits for a Risk or Prevalence

Using this formula with the example of 20 cases of influenza in 100 people, we can calculate the lower bound of a 90% confidence interval for the risk as follows.

$$R_L = R - Z \cdot \text{SE}(R) = 0.20 - 1.645 \cdot \sqrt{\frac{20 \cdot 80}{100^3}} = 0.13$$

The upper bound could be obtained by substituting a plus sign for the minus sign in the above calculation. Making this substitution gives a value of 0.27 for the upper bound. Thus, with 20 influenza cases in a population of 100 at risk, the 90% confidence interval for the risk estimate of 0.2 is 0.13–0.27.

Wilson's confidence limits for a binomial

The application of the preceding formula to risk data to obtain confidence limits is straightforward, but the approach is useful only as a large-number approximation. With scanty data, and especially for risks that are considerably less than (or greater than) 50%, the confidence limits are apt to be inaccurate. Suppose we have 20 people, among whom there is one case, for a risk estimate of 1/20 or 0.05. The text formula on page 131 would give a 90% confidence interval from -0.03 to 0.13. The lower limit is a negative risk, which does not even make sense. The lower limit should theoretically never go below 0, and the upper limit should never go above 1. These numbers are too small to use the binomial standard error formula. Because the risk estimate for this example is 0.05, there is less room for the risk to vary in the low direction than in the high direction, and an exact calculation of the confidence interval would produce limits that were not symmetrically placed around 0.05. The exact procedure, a more complicated calculation that goes beyond the scope of this book, gives a 90% confidence interval of 0.005–0.19. There is an approximate approach that comes close to exact limits for a binomial distribution, however. The formula was proposed in 1927 by Wilson:[1]

$$\frac{N}{N + Z^2}\left[\frac{a}{N} + \frac{Z^2}{2N} \pm Z\sqrt{\frac{a(N-a)}{N^3} + \frac{Z^2}{4N^2}}\right]$$

As before, a is the number of cases (numerator), N is the number at risk (denominator), and Z is the multiplier from the standard normal distribution that corresponds to the confidence level. This formula, much easier than an exact calculation, gives a 90% confidence interval for risk of 0.01–0.20, close to the exact confidence limits even for these small numbers. With this formula, there is little reason to obtain an exact binomial confidence interval for any data.

Incidence Rate Data

For incidence rate data, let us use a to represent cases and PT to represent person-time. Although the notation is similar to that for risk data, these data differ both conceptually and statistically from the binomial model used to describe risk data. For binomial data, the number of cases cannot exceed the total number of people at risk. In contrast, for rate data, the denominator does not relate to a specific number of people but rather to a time total. We do not know from the value of the person-time denominator, PT, how many people might have contributed time. For statistical purposes, we invoke a model for incidence rate data that allows the number of cases to vary without any upper limit. It is the Poisson model. We take a/PT as our estimate of the disease rate and calculate a confidence interval for the rate using formula 7–1 with the following standard error.

$$ SE(R) = \sqrt{\frac{a}{PT^2}} $$

Do rates always describe population samples?

Some theoreticians propose that if a rate or risk is measured in an entire population, there is no point in calculating a confidence interval, because a confidence interval is intended to convey only the imprecision that comes from taking a sample from a population. According to this reasoning, if one measures the entire population instead of a sample, there is no sampling error to worry about and, therefore, no confidence interval to compute. There is another side to this argument, however: others hold that even if the rate or risk is measured in an entire population, that population represents only a sample of people from a hypothetical superpopulation. In other words, the study population, even if enumerated completely without any sampling, represents merely a biologic sample of a larger set of people; therefore, a confidence interval is justified.

The validity of each argument may depend on the context. If one is measuring voter preference, it is the actual population in which one is interested, and the first argument is reasonable. For biologic phenomena, however, what happens in an actual population may be of less interest than the biologic norm that describes the super-population; therefore, the second argument is more compelling.

Example: Confidence Limits for an Incidence Rate

Consider as an example a cancer incidence rate estimated from a registry that reports 8 cases of astrocytoma among 85,000 person-years at risk. The rate is 8/85,000 person-years or 9.4 cases per 100,000 person-years. A lower 90% confidence limit for the rate would be estimated as follows.

$$ R_L = R - Z \cdot SE(R) = \frac{8}{85{,}000 \text{ person-years}} - 1.645 \cdot \sqrt{\frac{8}{(85{,}000 \text{ person-years})^2}} $$

$$ = 3.9 \text{ / } 100{,}000 \text{ person-years} $$

Using the plus sign instead of the minus sign in the above expression gives 14.9/100,000 person-years for the upper bound.

Byar's confidence limits

With very small numbers, the approximate formula given in the text for confidence limits for incidence rate data will be inaccurate. Once again, the ideal would be to calculate exact confidence limits, but as for risk data, there is also a convenient approximate formula that is nearly as good as exact methods and much easier to use. This formula, adapted from D. Byar (unpublished), is:

$$R_L, R_U = \frac{a' \cdot \left(1 - \frac{1}{9a'} \pm \frac{Z}{3}\sqrt{\frac{1}{a'}}\right)^3}{PT}$$

where a' equals $a + 0.5$, PT is the rate denominator, and Z is the multiplier from the standard normal distribution that corresponds to the level of confidence. As before, the minus sign is used to calculate the lower limit and the plus sign, the upper limit.

Suppose that the observed rate were 3 cases in 2500 person-years, for a rate of 12 cases per 10,000 person-years. The large-number formula for confidence limits in the text gives a symmetric 90% confidence interval of 0.6–23 cases per 10,000 person-years, whereas the above formula gives a 90% confidence interval of 4.3–28 cases per 10,000 person-years, which is much more accurate. (The exact confidence limits are 4.0 and 29.) Like Wilson's binomial formula and the exact confidence interval, the Byar confidence interval is asymmetrical.

Confidence Intervals for Measures of Effect

Studies that measure the effect of an exposure involve comparison of two or more groups. Cohort studies may be conducted using a fixed follow-up period for each person, obtaining effect estimates from a comparison of risk data; or they may allow for varying follow-up times for each person, obtaining effect estimates from a comparison of incidence rate data. Case-control studies come in several varieties, depending on how the controls are sampled; but for the most part, the analysis of case-control studies is based on a single underlying statistical model that describes the statistical behavior of the odds ratio. Prevalence data, obtained from surveys or cross-sectional studies, may usually be treated as risk data for statistical analysis because, like risk data, they represent proportions. Similarly, case fatality rates, which are more aptly described as data on risk of death among those with a given disease, may usually be considered risk data.

Cohort Studies with Risk Data (or Prevalence Data)

Consider a cohort study of a dichotomous exposure with the categories exposed and unexposed. If the study followed all subjects for a fixed period of time and there were no important competing risks and no confounding, we could display the essential data as follows.

	Exposed	Unexposed
Cases	a	b
People at risk	N_1	N_0

From this array, one can easily estimate the risk difference, *RD*, and the risk ratio, *RR*.

$$RD = \frac{a}{N_1} - \frac{b}{N_0}$$

$$RR = \frac{a}{N_1} \bigg/ \frac{b}{N_0}$$

To apply formulas 6–1 and 6–2 to obtain confidence intervals for the risk difference and the risk ratio, we need formulas for the standard error of *RD* and the ln(*RR*):

$$SE(RD) = \sqrt{\frac{a(N_1 - a)}{N_1^3} + \frac{b(N_0 - b)}{N_0^3}} \tag{7-2}$$

$$SE[\ln(RR)] = \sqrt{\frac{1}{a} - \frac{1}{N_1} + \frac{1}{b} - \frac{1}{N_0}} \tag{7-3}$$

Example: Confidence Limits for Risk Difference and Risk Ratio

As an example of risk data, consider Table 7–1, which describes recurrence risks among women with breast cancer treated with either tamoxifen or a combination of tamoxifen and radiotherapy.

Table 7–1. Risk of recurrence of breast cancer in a randomized trial of women treated with tamoxifen and radiotherapy or tamoxifen alone*

	Tamoxifen and Radiotherapy	Tamoxifen Only
Women with recurrence	321	411
Total women treated	686	689

*Data from Overgaard et al.[2]

From the data in Table 7–1, we can calculate a risk of recurrence of $321/686 = 0.47$ among women treated with tamoxifen and radiotherapy and a risk of $411/689 = 0.60$ among women treated with tamoxifen alone. The risk difference is $0.47 - 0.60 = -0.13$, with the minus sign indicating that the treatment group receiving both tamoxifen and radio-therapy had the lower risk. To obtain a 90% confidence interval for this estimate of risk difference, we use formulas 6–1 and 7–2 as follows.

$$RD_L = -0.13 - 1.645 \cdot \sqrt{\frac{321 \cdot 365}{686^3} + \frac{411 \cdot 278}{689^3}}$$

$$= -0.13 - 1.645 \cdot 0.027 = -0.17$$

$$RD_U = -0.13 + 1.645 \cdot \sqrt{\frac{321 \cdot 365}{686^3} + \frac{411 \cdot 278}{689^3}}$$

$$= -0.13 + 1.645 \cdot 0.027 = -0.08$$

This calculation gives 90% confidence limits around -0.13 of -0.17 and -0.08. In other words, the 90% confidence interval for the risk differ-ence ranges from a benefit of 17% smaller risk to a benefit of 8% smaller risk for women receiving the combined tamoxifen and radiotherapy treatment.

We can also compute the risk ratio and its confidence interval from the same data. The risk ratio is $(321/686)/(411/689) = 0.78$, indicating that the group receiving combined treatment faces a risk of recurrence that is 22% lower $(1 - 0.78)$ relative to the risk of recurrence among women receiving tamoxifen alone. The 90% lower confidence bound for the risk ratio is calculated as follows.

$$RR_L = e^{\ln(0.78) - 1.645 \cdot \sqrt{\frac{1}{321} - \frac{1}{686} + \frac{1}{411} - \frac{1}{689}}}$$

$$= e^{-0.24 - 1.645 \cdot 0.051} = e^{-0.327} = 0.72$$

Substituting a plus sign for the minus sign before the z-multiplier of 1.645 gives 0.85 for the upper limit. Thus, the 90% confidence interval for the risk ratio estimate of 0.78 is 0.72–0.85. In other words, the 90% confidence interval for this benefit of combined treatment ranges from a 28% lower risk to a 15% lower risk. (It is common when describing a reduced risk to convert the risk ratio to a relative decrease in risk by subtracting it from unity; thus, a lower limit for the risk ratio equal to 0.72 indicates a 28% lower risk because $1 - 0.72 = 0.28$, or 28%.) These percentages indicate a risk measured in relation to the risk among those receiving tamoxifen alone: the 28% lower limit refers to a risk that is 28% lower than the risk among those receiving tamoxifen alone.

Confidence intervals versus confidence limits

A *confidence interval* is a range of values about a point estimate that indicates the degree of statistical precision that describes the estimate. The level of confidence is set arbitrarily, but for any given level of confidence, the width of the interval expresses the precision of the measurement: a wider interval implies less precision, and a narrower interval implies more precision. The upper and lower boundaries of the interval are the *confidence limits*.

Cohort Studies with Incidence Rate Data

For cohort studies that measure incidence rates, we use the following notation.

	Exposed	Unexposed
Cases	a	b
Person-time at risk	PT_1	PT_0

The incidence rate among the exposed is a/PT_1 and that among the unexposed is b/PT_0. To obtain confidence intervals for the incidence rate difference (ID), $a/PT_1 - b/PT_0$, and the incidence rate ratio (IR), $(a/PT_1)/(b/PT_0)$, we use the following formulas for the standard error of the rate difference and the logarithm of the incidence rate ratio.

$$\text{SE}(ID) = \sqrt{\frac{a}{PT_1{}^2} + \frac{b}{PT_0{}^2}} \qquad (7\text{--}4)$$

$$\text{SE}[\ln(IR)] = \sqrt{\frac{1}{a} + \frac{1}{b}} \qquad (7\text{--}5)$$

Example: Confidence Limits for Incidence Rate Difference and Incidence Rate Ratio

The data in Table 7–2 are taken from a study by Feychting et al.,[3] comparing cancer occurrence among the blind with occurrence among those who were not blind but had severe visual impairment. (The study hypothesis was that a high circulating level of melatonin protects against cancer; melatonin production is greater among the blind because, among those who see, visual detection of light suppresses melatonin production by the pineal gland.)

Table 7–2. Incidence rate of cancer among a blind population and a population that is severely visually impaired but not blind*

	Blind	**Severely Visually Impaired but Not Blind**
Cancer cases	136	1709
Person-years	22,050	127,650

*Data from Feychting et al.[3]

From these data we can calculate a cancer rate of 136/22,050 person-years = 6.2/1000 person-years among the blind compared with 1709/127,650 person-years = 13.4/1000 person-years among those who were visually impaired but not blind. The incidence rate difference is (6.2 − 13.4)/1000 person-years = −7.2/1000 person-years. The minus sign indicates that the rate is lower among the group with total blindness, which is here considered the "exposed" group. To obtain a 90% confidence interval for this estimate of rate difference, we use formula 6–1 in combination with formula 7–4, as follows.

$$ID_L = \frac{-7.2}{1000 \text{ person-years}} - 1.645 \cdot \sqrt{\frac{136}{22,050^2} + \frac{1709}{127,650^2}}$$

$$= \frac{-7.2}{1000 \text{ person-years}} - 1.645 \cdot \frac{0.62}{1000 \text{ person-years}} = \frac{-8.2}{1000 \text{ person-years}}$$

$$ID_U = \frac{-7.2}{1000 \text{ person-years}} + 1.645 \cdot \sqrt{\frac{136}{22,050^2} + \frac{1709}{127,650^2}}$$

$$= \frac{-7.2}{1000 \text{ person-years}} + 1.645 \cdot \frac{0.62}{1000 \text{ person-years}} = \frac{-6.2}{1000 \text{ person-years}}$$

This calculation gives 90% confidence limits around the rate difference of −7.2/1000 person-years of −8.2/1000 person-years and −6.2/1000 person-years.

The incidence rate ratio for the data in Table 7–2 is (136/22,050)/(1709/127,650) = 0.46, indicating a rate among the blind that is less than half that among the comparison group. The lower limit of the 90% confidence interval for this rate ratio is calculated as follows.

$$IR_L = e^{\ln(0.46) - 1.645 \cdot \sqrt{\frac{1}{136} + \frac{1}{1709}}}$$

$$= e^{-0.775 - 1.645 \cdot 0.089} = e^{-0.922} = 0.40$$

A corresponding calculation for the upper limit gives $IR_U = 0.53$, for a 90% confidence interval around the incidence rate ratio of 0.46 of 0.40–0.53.

Case-Control Studies

Here and in later chapters we deal with methods for the analysis of a density case-control study, the most common form of case-control study. The analysis of case-cohort studies and case-crossover studies is slightly different and is left for more advanced texts. For the data display from a case-control study, we will use the following notation.

	Exposed	Unexposed
Cases	a	b
Controls	c	d

The primary estimate of effect that we can derive from these data is the incidence rate ratio, which in case-control studies is estimated from the odds ratio (OR), ad/bc. We obtain an approximate confidence interval for the odds ratio using the following formula for the standard error of the logarithm of the odds ratio:

$$SE[\ln(OR)] = \sqrt{\frac{1}{a} + \frac{1}{b} + \frac{1}{c} + \frac{1}{d}} \qquad (7\text{--}6)$$

Example: Confidence Limits for the Odds Ratio

Consider as an example the data in Table 7–3 on amphetamine use and stroke in young women, from the study by Petitti et al.[3]

For these case-control data, we can calculate an OR of $(10)(1016)/[(5)(337)] = 6.0$. An approximate 90% confidence interval for this odds ratio can be calculated from the standard error expression 7–6 above in combination with formula 6–1.

$$OR_L = e^{\ln(6.0) - 1.645 \cdot \sqrt{\frac{1}{10} + \frac{1}{337} + \frac{1}{5} + \frac{1}{1016}}}$$

$$= e^{1.797 - 1.645 \cdot 0.551} = e^{1.797 - 0.907} = e^{0.890} = 2.4$$

Table 7–3. Frequency of recent amphetamine use among stroke cases and controls among women age 15–44*

	Amphetamine Use	No Amphetamine Use
Stroke cases	10	337
Controls	5	1016

*Adapted from Petitti et al.[4]

Using a plus sign instead of the minus sign in front of the z-multiplier of
1.645, we get $OR_U = 14.9$. The point estimate of 6.0 for the odds ratio is
the geometric mean between the lower limit and the upper limit of the
confidence interval. This relation applies whenever we set confidence
intervals on the log scale, which we do for all approximate intervals for
ratio measures. The limits are symmetrically placed about the point estimate on the log scale, but the upper bound appears farther from the
point estimate on the untransformed ratio scale. This asymmetry on the
untransformed scale for a ratio measure is especially apparent in this
example because the OR estimate is large.

Calculation of *p* Values

Although the reader is better off relying on estimation rather than tests
of statistical significance for inference, for completeness we give here the
basic formulas from which traditional *p* values can be derived that test
the null hypothesis that exposure is not related to disease.

Risk Data

For risk data, we will use the following expansion of the notation used
earlier in the chapter.

	Exposed	Unexposed	Total
Cases	a	b	M_1
Noncases	c	d	M_0
People at risk	N_1	N_0	T

The *p* value testing the null hypothesis that exposure is not related to
disease can be obtained from the following formula for χ.

$$\chi = \frac{a - \dfrac{N_1 M_1}{T}}{\sqrt{\dfrac{N_1 N_0 M_1 M_0}{T^2 (T-1)}}} \tag{7-7}$$

For the data in Table 7–1, formula 7–7 gives χ as follows.

$$\chi = \frac{321 - \dfrac{686 \cdot 732}{1375}}{\sqrt{\dfrac{686 \cdot 689 \cdot 732 \cdot 643}{1375^2 \cdot 1374}}} = \frac{321 - 365.20}{\sqrt{85.64}} = -4.78$$

The *p* value that corresponds to the χ statistic must be obtained from
tables of the standard normal distribution (see Appendix). For a χ of

−4.78 (the minus sign indicates only that the exposed group had a lower risk than the unexposed group), the p value is very small (roughly 0.0000009). The Appendix tabulates values of χ only from −3.99 to +3.99.

Incidence Rate Data

For incidence rate data, we use the following notation, which is an expanded version of the table we used earlier:

	Exposed	Unexposed	Total
Cases	a	b	M
Person-time	PT_1	PT_0	T

We can use the following formula to calculate χ.

$$\chi = \frac{a - \dfrac{PT_1}{T} M}{\sqrt{M \dfrac{PT_1}{T} \dfrac{PT_0}{T}}} \tag{7-8}$$

Applying this formula to the data of Table 7–2 gives the following result for χ.

$$\chi = \frac{136 - \dfrac{22{,}050 \cdot 1845}{149{,}700}}{\sqrt{1845 \cdot \dfrac{22{,}050}{149{,}700} \cdot \dfrac{127{,}650}{149{,}700}}} = \frac{136 - 271.76}{\sqrt{231.73}} = -8.92$$

This χ is so large in absolute value that the p value cannot be readily calculated. The p value corresponding to a χ of −8.92 is much smaller than 10^{-20}, implying that the data are not readily consistent with a chance explanation.

Case-Control Data

For case-control data, we can apply formula 7–7 to the data in Table 7–3.

$$\chi = \frac{10 - \dfrac{15 \cdot 347}{1368}}{\sqrt{\dfrac{15 \cdot 1353 \cdot 347 \cdot 1021}{1368^2 \cdot 1367}}} = \frac{10 - 3.80}{\sqrt{2.81}} = -3.70$$

This result corresponds to a p value of 0.00022.

Questions

1. With person-time data, the numerators are considered Poisson random variables and the denominators are treated as if they were constants, not subject to variability. In fact, however, the person-time must be measured and is therefore subject to measurement error. Why are the denominators treated as constants if they are subject to measurement error? What would be the effect on the confidence interval of taking this measurement error into account instead of ignoring it?
2. The usual approximate formula for confidence limits for risk or prevalence data, based on the binomial distribution, will not work if there are zero cases in the numerator. The Wilson formula, however, is still useful in such situations. It gives zero for the lower limit, which is appropriate, and it gives a meaningful upper limit. Suppose that you were interested in the case fatality rate among patients undergoing bypass cardiac surgery in a new cardiac surgery unit. Among the first 30 patients to undergo surgery, none died within 30 days. Using the Wilson formula, calculate a 90% confidence interval for the risk of dying within 30 days after surgery.
3. Why do you suppose that the estimation formulas to obtain confidence intervals are the same for prevalence data and risk data (formulas 7–2 and 7–3)?
4. Why do you suppose that the estimation formulas for confidence intervals differ for risk data and case-control data (formulas 7–3 and 7–6) but the formula for obtaining a χ statistic to test the null hypothesis is the same for risk data and case-control data (formula 7–7)?
5. Does it lend a false sense of precision if one presents a 90% confidence interval instead of a 95% confidence interval?
6. Calculate a 90% confidence interval and a 95% confidence interval for the odds ratio from the following crude case-control data relating to the effect of exposure to magnetic fields on risk of acute leukemia in children.[5]

	Median night-time exposure		
	≥2 μT	<2 μT	Total
Cases	9	167	176
Controls	5	409	414
Total	14	576	590

References

1. Wilson EB: Probable inference. The law of succession and statistical inference. *J Amer Stat Assn* 1927; 22:209–212.
2. Overgaard, M, Jensen, M-B, Overgaard, J, et al: Postoperative radiotherapy in high-risk postmenopausal breast-cancer patients given adju-

vant tamoxifen: Danish Breast Cancer Cooperative Group DBCG 82c randomised trial. *Lancet* 1999;353:1641–1648.

3. Feychting, M, Osterlund, B, Ahlbom, A. Reduced cancer incidence among the blind. *Epidemiology* 1998;9:490–494.

4. Petitti, DB, Sidney, S, Quesenberry, C, et al: Stroke and cocaine or amphetamine use. *Epidemiology* 1998;9:596–600.

5. Michaelis, J, Schuz, J, Meinert, R, et al: Combined risk estimates for two German population-based case-control studies on residential magnetic fields and childhood acute leukemia. *Epidemiology* 1998;9:92–94.

8

Controlling Confounding by Stratifying Data

Earlier we saw that the apparent effect of birth order on the prevalence at birth of Down syndrome (Fig. 5–2) is attributable to confounding. As demonstrated in Figure 5–3, maternal age has an extremely strong relation to the prevalence of Down syndrome. In Figure 5–4, which classifies the Down syndrome data simultaneously by birth order and maternal age, we can see that there is a maternal-age effect at every level of birth order, but no clear birth-order effect at any level of maternal age. The birth-order effect in the crude data is confounded by maternal age, which is correlated with birth order.

Figure 5–4 is a graphic demonstration of *stratification. Stratification* is basically the cross-tabulation of data; usually, stratification refers to cross-tabulation of data on exposure and disease by categories of one or more other variables that are potential confounding variables. We saw another example of stratification in Chapter 1, which introduced the concept of confounding. Stratification is an effective and straightforward means to control confounding. In this chapter, we explore stratification in greater detail and present simple formulas to derive an unconfounded estimate of an effect from stratified data.

An Example of Confounding

First, let us consider another example of confounding. The data in Table 8–1 are mortality rates for male and female patients with trigeminal neuralgia, a recurrent paroxysmal pain of the face. The rate ratio of 1.10 indicates a slightly greater mortality rate for males than for females in these crude data. (The male group may be thought of as the "exposed" group and the female group as the "unexposed" group, to make this example analogous to other settings in which the "exposure" variable is a specific agent.) This estimate of the effect of being male on the death rate of trigeminal neuralgia patients is confounded, however. Table 8–2 shows the data stratified into two age groups, split at age 65. The age stratification reveals several interesting things about the data. First, as

Table 8-1. Mortality rates among patients with trigeminal neuralgia, by sex*

	Males	**Females**
Deaths	90	131
Person-years	2465	3946
Mortality rate	36.5/1000 person-years	33.2/1000 person-years
Rate ratio		1.10
90% CI		0.88–1.38

*Data from Rothman and Monson.[1]

one might predict, patients in the older age group have much higher death rates than those in the younger age group. The striking increase in risk of death with age is typical of any population of older adults, even adults in the general population. Second, the stratification shows a difference in the age distribution of the person-time of male and female patients: the male person-time is mainly in the under 65 category, whereas the female person-time is predominantly in the 65 or older category. Thus, the female experience is older than the male experience. This age difference would tend to produce a lower overall death rate in males relative to females, because to some extent comparing the death rate among males with that among females is a comparison of young with old. Third, in the crude data, the rate ratio (male/female) was 1.10 but in the two age categories it was 1.57 and 1.49, respectively. This discrepancy between the crude rate ratio and the rate ratios for each of the two age categories is a result of the strong age effect and the fact that female patients tend to be older than male patients. It is a good example of confounding by age, in this case biasing the crude rate ratio downward because the male person-time experience is younger than that of the females.

Table 8-2. Mortality rates among patients with trigeminal neuralgia, by sex and age category*

	Age (years)			
	<65		**≥65**	
	Males	**Females**	**Males**	**Females**
Deaths	14	10	76	121
Person-years	1516	1701	949	2245
Mortality rate (cases/1000 person-years)	9.2	5.9	80.1	53.9
Rate ratio	1.57		1.49	

*Data from Rothman and Monson.[1]

Stratification into age categories allows us to assess the presence of confounding. It also permits us to refine the estimate of the rate ratio by controlling age confounding. Below, we use this trigeminal neuralgia example and examples of other types of data to obtain unconfounded effect estimates using stratification.

Unconfounded Effect Estimates and Confidence Intervals from Stratified Data

How does stratification control confounding? Confounding, as explained in Chapter 5, comes from the mixing of the effect of the confounding variable with the effect of the exposure. If a variable that is a risk factor for the disease is associated with the exposure in the study population, confounding will result. Confounding comes about because the comparison of exposed with unexposed people is also a comparison of those with differing distributions of the confounding factor: in the trigeminal neuralgia example above, comparing men with women was also a comparison of younger people (the men in the study) with older people (the women in the study). Stratification creates subgroups in which the confounding factor either does not vary at all or does not vary much. Stratification by nominal scale variables, such as sex or country of birth, theoretically results in strata in which the variables of sex or country of birth do not vary; in actuality, there may still be some residual variability because some people may be misclassified into the wrong strata. Stratification by a continuously measured variable, such as age, will result in age categories within which age can vary, but over a restricted range. With either kind of variable, nominal scale or continuous, a stratified analysis proceeds under the assumption that within the categories of the stratification variable there is no meaningful variability of the potential confounding factor. If the stratification variable is continuous, like age, then the more categories that are used to form strata, the less variability by age there will be within those categories.

A stratified analysis can be as straightforward as a presentation of the data within each of the strata. Often, however, the investigator hopes to summarize the relation between exposure and disease in a simple way. The way to do that is to make the essential comparisons within each stratum and then to aggregate the information from these comparisons over all strata. There are two methods to aggregate the information over strata, *pooling* and *standardization,* each with its own formula for combining the data across strata.

Pooling

Pooling is one method for obtaining unconfounded estimates of effect across a set of strata. When pooling is used, it comes with an important assumption: that the effect being estimated is constant across the strata.

With this assumption, one can view each stratum as providing a separate estimate (referred to as a *stratum-specific estimate*) of the overall effect. With each stratum providing a separate estimate of effect, the principle behind pooling is simply to take an average of these stratum-specific estimates of effect. The average is taken as a weighted average, which is a method of averaging that assigns more weight to some values than others. In pooling, weights are assigned so that the strata providing the most information, that is, the strata with the most data, get the most weight. In the formulas presented below, this weighting is built directly into the calculations. When the data do not conform to the assumption necessary for pooling that the effect is constant across all strata, pooling is not applicable. In such a situation, it is still possible to obtain an unconfounded summary estimate of the effect over the strata using *standardization,* which is discussed later in this chapter.

Cohort Studies with Risk Data (or Prevalence Data)

Let us consider risk data. (Prevalence data may be treated the same as risk data.) We use the same basic notation as we did for unstratified data, but we add a stratum-identifying subscript, i, which ranges from 1 to the total number of strata. The notation for stratum i in a set of strata of risk data would be as follows.

	Exposed	Unexposed	Total
Cases	a_i	b_i	M_{1i}
Noncases	c_i	d_i	M_{0i}
Total at risk	N_{1i}	N_{0i}	T_i

For risk data, we can calculate a pooled estimate of the risk difference or the risk ratio. The pooled risk difference may be estimated from stratified data using the following formula.

$$RD_{\text{MH}} = \frac{\sum_i \dfrac{a_i N_{0i} - b_i N_{1i}}{T_i}}{\sum_i \dfrac{N_{1i} N_{0i}}{T_i}} \tag{8-1}$$

Σ signifies summation over all values of the stratum indicator i. The subscript *MH* for the pooled risk difference measure refers to 'Mantel-Haenszel,' indicating that the formula is one of a group of formulas for pooled estimates that derive from an approach originally introduced by Mantel and Haenszel.[2]

The formula for the pooled risk ratio from stratified risk or prevalence data is as follows:

$$RR_{\mathrm{MH}} = \frac{\sum_i \dfrac{a_i N_{0i}}{T_i}}{\sum_i \dfrac{b_i N_{1i}}{T_i}} \tag{8-2}$$

Example: Stratification of Risk Data

To illustrate the stratification of risk data, let us revisit the example of the University Group Diabetes Program (Tables 5–3 and 5–4). For convenience, the age-specific data are repeated here in Table 8–3. First, we consider the risk difference. From the crude data, the risk difference is 4.5%. Contrary to expectations, the tolbutamide group experienced a greater risk of death than the placebo group, despite the fact that tolbutamide was thought to prevent complications of diabetes that might lead to death. Critics of the study believed this finding to be erroneous and looked for explanations such as confounding. Age was one of the possible confounding factors. By chance, the tolbutamide group tended to be slightly older than the placebo group. This age difference is evident in Table 8–3: 48% (98/204) of the tolbutamide group is at least 55 years of age, whereas only 41% (85/205) of the placebo group is at least 55 years of age. We know that older people have a greater risk of death, a relation that is also evident in Table 8–3. Consider the placebo group: the risk of death during the study period was 18.8% for the older age group but only 4.2% for the younger age group. Therefore, we would suspect that the greater risk of death in the tolbutamide group is in part due to confounding by age. We can explore this issue further by obtaining a pooled estimate of the risk difference for tolbutamide compared with placebo after stratifying by the two age strata in Table 8–3.

Table 8–3. Risk of death for groups receiving tolbutamide or placebo in the University Group Diabetes Program, overall and by age category (1970)*

	Age				Total	
	<55		≥55			
	Tolb	Placebo	Tolb	Placebo	Tolb	Placebo
Deaths	8	5	22	16	30	21
Total at risk	106	120	98	85	204	205
Risk of death	0.076	0.042	0.224	0.188	0.147	0.102
Risk difference	0.034		0.036		0.045	
Risk ratio	1.81		1.19		1.44	

*Data from the University Group Diabetes Program.[3]

We obtain a pooled estimate of the risk difference by applying formula 8–1, as follows.

$$RD_{MH} = \frac{\dfrac{8 \cdot 120 - 5 \cdot 106}{226} + \dfrac{22 \cdot 85 - 16 \cdot 98}{183}}{\dfrac{106 \cdot 120}{226} + \dfrac{98 \cdot 85}{183}} = \frac{1.903 + 1.650}{56.283 + 45.519} = 0.035$$

The result, 3.5%, is smaller than the risk difference in the crude data, 4.5%. Note that 3.5% is within the narrow range of the two stratum-specific risk differences in Table 8–3, 3.4% for age <55 and 3.6% for age ≥55. Mathematically, the pooled estimate is a weighted average of the stratum-specific values, so it will always be within the range of the stratum-specific estimates of the effect. The crude estimate of effect, however, is not within this range. We should regard the 3.5% as a more appropriate estimate than the estimate from the crude data, as it removes age confounding. The crude risk difference differs from the unconfounded estimate because the crude estimate reflects not only the effect of tolbutamide (which we estimate to be 3.5% from this analysis) but also the confounding effect of age. Because the tolbutamide group is older on average than the placebo group, the risk difference in the crude data is greater than the unconfounded risk difference. If the tolbutamide group had been younger than the placebo group, then the confounding would have worked in the opposite direction, resulting in a lower risk difference in the crude data than from the pooled analysis after stratification.

The unconfounded estimate of risk difference, 3.5%, is unconfounded only to the extent that stratification into these two broad age categories removes age confounding. It is likely that some residual confounding remains (see box) and that the risk difference unconfounded by age is smaller than 3.5%.

We can also calculate a pooled estimate of the risk ratio from the data in Table 8–3, using formula 8–2.

$$RR_{MH} = \frac{\dfrac{8 \cdot 120}{226} + \dfrac{22 \cdot 85}{183}}{\dfrac{5 \cdot 106}{226} + \dfrac{16 \cdot 98}{183}} = \frac{4.248 + 10.219}{2.345 + 8.568} = 1.33$$

This result, like that for the risk difference, is closer to the null value than the crude risk ratio of 1.44, indicating that age confounding has been removed by the stratification. Once again, the pooled estimate is

---

Residual confounding

The two age categories in Table 8–3 may not be sufficient to control all of the age confounding in the data. In general, more strata, with narrower boundaries, will control confounding more effectively than fewer strata with broader boundaries. If age strata (or strata by any continuous stratification factor) are broad, there may be confounding within them. A stratified analysis controls only between-stratum confounding, not within-stratum confounding. Within-stratum confounding is often referred to as *residual confounding*. The same term is used to describe confounding from factors that are not controlled at all in a study or from factors that are controlled but are measured inaccurately from the beginning.

To avoid within-stratum residual confounding, it is desirable to carve the data into more strata and to avoid open-ended strata (such as age ≥55) when possible. On the other hand, stratifying too finely may stretch the data unreasonably, producing small frequencies of events within cells and leading to imprecise results. Finding the best number of strata to use in a given analysis often requires balancing the need to control confounding against the need to avoid random error in the estimation, and ends up being a compromise.

---

within the range of the stratum-specific estimates, as it must be. Note, however, that for the risk ratio, the stratum-specific estimates for the data in Table 8–3, 1.81 and 1.19, differ considerably from one another. The wide range between them includes not only the pooled estimate but also the estimate of effect from the crude data. When the stratum-specific estimates of effect are nearly identical, as they were for the risk differences in the data in Table 8–3, we have a good idea of what the pooled estimate will be just from inspecting the stratum-specific data. When the stratum-specific estimates vary, it will not be as clear on inspection what the pooled estimate will be.

As stated above, the formulas to obtain pooled estimates are premised on the assumption that the effect is constant across strata. Thus, the pooled risk ratio of 1.33 for the above example is premised on the assumption that there is a single value for the risk ratio that applies to both the young and the old strata. This assumption seems reasonable for the risk difference calculation, for which the two strata gave nearly the same estimate of risk difference; but how can we use this assumption to estimate the risk ratio when the two age strata give such different risk ratio estimates? The assumption does not imply that the estimates of effect will be the same, or even nearly the same, in each stratum. It allows for statistical variation over the strata. It is possible to conduct a statistical evaluation, called either a *test of heterogeneity* or a *test of homo-*

geneity, to determine whether the variation in estimates from one stratum to another is compatible with the assumption that the effect is uniform.[4] In any event, it is helpful to keep in mind that the assumption that the effect is uniform is probably wrong in most situations. It is asking too much to have the effect be absolutely constant over the categories of some stratification factor. It is more realistic to consider the assumption as a fictional convenience, one that facilitates the computation of a pooled estimate. Unless the data demonstrate some clear pattern of variation that undermines the assumption that the effect is uniform over the strata, it is usually reasonable to use a pooled approach, despite the fiction of the assumption. In Table 8–3, the variation of the risk ratio estimates for the two age strata is not striking enough to warrant concern about the assumption that the risk ratio is uniform. If one undertakes a more formal statistical evaluation of the assumption of uniformity for these data, it would support the view that the assumption of a uniform risk ratio for the data in Table 8–3 is reasonable.

Confidence Intervals for Pooled Estimates

To obtain confidence intervals for the pooled estimates of effect, we need variance formulas to combine with the point estimates. Table 8–4 lists variance formulas for the various pooled estimates that we consider in this chapter.

Although the formulas look complicated, they are easy to apply. Each variance formula corresponds to a particular type of stratified data. First, consider the pooled risk difference. For the data in Table 8–3, we calculated that RD_{MH} was 0.035. We can derive the variance for this estimate, and thus a confidence interval, by applying the first formula from Table 8–4 to the data in Table 8–3.

$Var(RD_{MH})$

$$= \frac{\left(\frac{106 \cdot 120}{226}\right)^2 \left(\frac{8 \cdot 98}{106^2 \cdot 105} + \frac{5 \cdot 115}{120^2 \cdot 119}\right) + \left(\frac{98 \cdot 85}{183}\right)^2 \left(\frac{22 \cdot 76}{98^2 \cdot 97} + \frac{16 \cdot 69}{85^2 \cdot 84}\right)}{\left[\left(\frac{106 \cdot 120}{226}\right) + \left(\frac{98 \cdot 85}{183}\right)\right]^2}$$

$$= \frac{3.1681 + 7.4879}{10,363.7} = 0.001028$$

This gives a standard error of $(0.001028)^{1/2} = 0.0321$ and a 90% confidence interval of $0.035 \pm 1.645 \cdot 0.0321 = 0.035 \pm 0.053 = -0.018$ to 0.088. The confidence interval is broad enough to indicate a fair amount of statistical uncertainty in the finding that tolbutamide is worse than placebo. Notably, however, the data are not compatible with any compelling benefit for tolbutamide.

Table 8–4. Variance formulas for pooled analyses

$$\text{Risk difference: } \mathrm{Var}(RD_{\mathrm{MH}}) = \frac{\displaystyle\sum_i \left(\frac{N_{1i}N_{0i}}{T_i}\right)^2 \left[\frac{a_i c_i}{N_{1i}^2\,(N_{1i}-1)} + \frac{b_i d_i}{N_{0i}^2\,(N_{0i}-1)}\right]}{\left(\displaystyle\sum_i \frac{N_{1i}N_{0i}}{T_i}\right)^2}$$

$$\text{Risk ratio: } \mathrm{Var}[\ln(RR_{\mathrm{MH}})] = \frac{\displaystyle\sum_i (M_{1i}N_{1i}N_{0i}/T_i^2 - a_i b_i/T_i)}{\left(\displaystyle\sum_i \frac{a_i N_{0i}}{T_i}\right)\left(\displaystyle\sum_i \frac{b_i N_{1i}}{T_i}\right)}$$

$$\text{Incidence rate difference: } \mathrm{Var}(ID_{\mathrm{MH}}) = \frac{\displaystyle\sum_i (PT_{1i}PT_{0i}/T_i)^2\,(a_i/PT_{1i}^2 + b_i/PT_{0i}^2)}{\left(\displaystyle\sum_i (PT_{1i}PT_{0i}/T_i)\right)^2}$$

$$\text{Incidence rate ratio: } \mathrm{Var}[\ln(IR_{\mathrm{MH}})] = \frac{\displaystyle\sum_i (M_{1i}PT_{1i}PT_{0i}/T_i^2)}{\left(\displaystyle\sum_i \frac{a_i PT_{0i}}{T_i}\right)\left(\displaystyle\sum_i \frac{b_i PT_{1i}}{T_i}\right)}$$

$$\text{Odds ratio: } \mathrm{Var}[\ln(OR_{\mathrm{MH}})] = \frac{\displaystyle\sum_i G_i P_i}{2\left(\displaystyle\sum_i G_i\right)^2} + \frac{\displaystyle\sum_i (G_i Q_i + H_i P_i)}{2\left(\displaystyle\sum_i G_i \sum_i H_i\right)} + \frac{\displaystyle\sum_i H_i Q_i}{2\left(\displaystyle\sum_i H_i\right)^2}$$

where
$G_i = (a_i d_i/T_i)$ $H_i = (b_i c_i/T_i)$
$P_i = (a_i + d_i)/T_i$ $Q_i = (b_i + c_i)/T_i$

One might also construct a confidence interval for the risk ratio estimated from the same stratified data. In that case, one would use the second formula in Table 8–4, setting limits on the log scale, as we did in the previous chapter for crude data.

$$\mathrm{Var}[\ln(RR_{\mathrm{MH}})] = \frac{\left(\dfrac{13\cdot 106\cdot 120}{226^2} - \dfrac{8\cdot 5}{226}\right) + \left(\dfrac{38\cdot 98\cdot 85}{183^2} - \dfrac{22\cdot 16}{183}\right)}{\left(\dfrac{8\cdot 120}{226} + \dfrac{22\cdot 85}{183}\right)\cdot\left(\dfrac{5\cdot 106}{226} + \dfrac{16\cdot 98}{183}\right)}$$

$$= \frac{3.0605 + 7.5286}{14.466\cdot 10.913} = \frac{10.5891}{157.88} = 0.0671$$

This result gives a standard error for the logarithm of the RR of $(0.0671)^{1/2}$ = 0.259 and a 90% confidence interval of 0.87–2.0.

$$RR_L = e^{\ln(1.33) - 1.645 \cdot 0.259} = 0.87$$

$$RR_U = e^{\ln(1.33) + 1.645 \cdot 0.259} = 2.0$$

The interpretation for this result is similar to that for the confidence interval of the risk difference, which is as one would expect since the two measures of effect and their respective confidence intervals are alternative ways of expressing the same finding from the same set of data.

As another example, consider again the data in Table 1–2. We can calculate the risk ratio for 20-year risk of death among smokers compared with nonsmokers across the seven age strata using formula 8–2. This calculation gives an overall Mantel-Haenszel risk ratio of 1.21, with a 90% confidence interval of 1.06–1.38. The Mantel-Haenszel risk ratio not only is different from the crude risk ratio of 0.76 but, as noted in Chapter 1, it points in the opposite direction.

Cohort Studies with Incidence Rate Data

For rate data, we have the following notation for stratum i of a stratified analysis.

	Exposed	Unexposed	Total
Cases	a_i	b_i	M_i
Person-time at risk	PT_{1i}	PT_{0i}	T_i

As for risk data, we can calculate a pooled estimate of the rate difference or the rate ratio. The pooled rate difference may be estimated from stratified data using the following formula.

$$ID_{MH} = \frac{\sum\limits_{i} \dfrac{a_i PT_{0i} - b_i PT_{1i}}{T_i}}{\sum\limits_{i} \dfrac{PT_{1i} PT_{0i}}{T_i}} \tag{8-4}$$

A pooled estimate of the rate ratio may be estimated as follows:

$$IR_{MH} = \frac{\sum\limits_{i} \dfrac{a_i PT_{0i}}{T_i}}{\sum\limits_{i} \dfrac{b_i PT_{1i}}{T_i}} \tag{8-5}$$

Table 8–5. Mortality rates for current and past clozapine users, overall and by age category*

	Age (years)					
	10–54		*55–94*		*Total*	
	Current	**Past**	**Current**	**Past**	**Current**	**Past**
Deaths	196	111	167	157	363	268
Person-years	62,119	15,763	6085	2780	68,204	18,543
Rate ($\times 10^5$ years)	315.5	704.2	2744	5647	532.2	1445
Rate difference ($\times 10^5$ years)	−388.7		−2903		−912.8	
Rate ratio	0.45		0.49		0.37	

*Data from Walker et al.[5]

As an illustration, consider the rate data in Table 8–5. These data come from a study of mortality rates among current users and past users of clozapine, a drug used to treat schizophrenia. As clozapine is thought to affect mortality primarily for current users, the experience of past users was used as the reference by which to judge the effect of current use. As for the tolbutamide example, the data are stratified into two broad age categories.

The death rates are much greater for older patients than for younger patients, as one would expect: among schizophrenia patients, just as for the general population, death rates climb strikingly with age. There is also an association between age and current versus past use of clozapine. Among current users, 9% (6085/68,204) of the person-time is in the older age category, whereas among past users 15% (2780/18,543) of the person-time is in the older age category. This difference is enough to introduce some confounding, although it is not large enough to produce more than a modest amount. Because the person-time for past use has an older age distribution, the age differences will lead to lower death rates among current users. The crude data do indicate a lower death rate among current users, with a rate difference of 912.8 cases per 100,000 person-years. At least some of this difference is attributable to age confounding. We can estimate the mortality rate difference that is unconfounded by age (apart from any residual age confounding within these broad age categories) from formula 8–4.

$$ID_{MH} = \frac{\dfrac{196 \cdot 15{,}763 - 111 \cdot 62{,}119}{77{,}882} + \dfrac{167 \cdot 2780 - 157 \cdot 6085}{8865}}{\dfrac{62{,}119 \cdot 15{,}763}{77{,}882} + \dfrac{6085 \cdot 2780}{8865}}$$

$$= \frac{-48.864 - 55.396}{12{,}572.633 + 1908.212} = -720.0 \times 10^{-5} \; \mathrm{yr}^{-1}$$

This result is smaller than the crude rate difference of -912.8×10^{-5} person-years, as was predictable from the direction of the difference in the age distributions. The amount of the confounding is modest, despite age being a strong risk factor, because the difference in the age distributions between current and past use is also modest. We cannot say that the remaining difference of -720.0×10^{-5} person-years is completely unconfounded by age because our age categorization comprises only two broad categories, but the pooled estimate removes some of the age confounding. Further control of age confounding might move the estimate further in the same direction, but it is unlikely that age confounding could account for the entire effect of current use on mortality.

What is the confidence interval for the pooled estimate? To obtain the interval, we use the third variance formula in Table 8–4.

$$\mathrm{Var}(ID_{\mathrm{MH}}) = \frac{\left(\dfrac{62{,}119 \cdot 15{,}763}{77{,}882}\right)^2 \left(\dfrac{196}{62{,}119^2} + \dfrac{111}{15{,}763^2}\right) + \left(\dfrac{6085 \cdot 780}{8865}\right)^2 \left(\dfrac{167}{6085^2} + \dfrac{157}{2780^2}\right)}{\left(\dfrac{62{,}119 \cdot 15{,}763}{77{,}882} + \dfrac{6085 \cdot 2780}{8865}\right)^2}$$

$$= \frac{78.644 + 90.394}{209{,}694{,}871.6} = 8.061 \times 10^{-7}$$

The square root of the variance gives a standard error of 89.8×10^{-5} person-years, for a 90% confidence interval of $(-720.0 \pm 1.645 \cdot 89.8) \times 10^{-5}$ person-years $= -867.7 \times 10^{-5}$ person-years, -572.3×10^{-5} person-years. The narrow confidence interval is the result of the large numbers of observations in the two strata.

The pooled incidence rate ratio for these same data is calculated from formula 8–5 as follows.

$$IR_{\mathrm{MH}} = \frac{\dfrac{196 \cdot 15{,}763}{77{,}882} + \dfrac{167 \cdot 2780}{8865}}{\dfrac{111 \cdot 62{,}119}{77{,}882} + \dfrac{157 \cdot 6085}{8865}} = \frac{39.67 + 52.37}{88.53 + 107.77} = 0.47$$

This value indicates that after control of confounding by age in these two age categories, current users have half the mortality rate of past users. (Note that we have been using the notation of incidence rate in the formulas, but we are actually describing mortality data. This use is legitimate because a mortality rate is an incidence rate of death.)

The 90% confidence interval for this pooled estimate of the mortality rate ratio can be calculated from the fourth variance formula in Table 8–4.

$$\text{Var}[\ln(IR_{\text{MH}})] = \frac{\dfrac{307 \cdot 62{,}119 \cdot 15{,}763}{77{,}882^2} + \dfrac{324 \cdot 6085 \cdot 2780}{8865^2}}{\left(\dfrac{196 \cdot 15{,}763}{77{,}882} + \dfrac{167 \cdot 2780}{8865}\right) \cdot \left(\dfrac{111 \cdot 62{,}119}{77{,}882} + \dfrac{157 \cdot 6085}{8865}\right)}$$

$$= \frac{49.56 + 69.74}{92.04 \cdot 196.30} = \frac{119.30}{18{,}067.4} = 0.00660$$

The corresponding standard error is $0.00660^{1/2} = 0.081$. The 90% confidence interval for the pooled rate ratio is calculated as follows:

$$IR_{\text{L}} = e^{\ln(0.47) - 1.645 \cdot 0.081} = 0.41$$

$$IR_{\text{U}} = e^{\ln(0.47) + 1.645 \cdot 0.081} = 0.54$$

This confidence interval is narrow, as is that for the rate difference, because there is a large number of deaths in the study. Thus, the study indicates with substantial precision that current users of clozapine had a much lower death rate than past users.

Case-Control Studies

For case-control data, we use the following notation for stratum i of a stratified analysis.

	Exposed	Unexposed	Total
Cases	a_i	b_i	M_{1i}
Controls	c_i	d_i	M_{0i}
Total	N_{1i}	N_{0i}	T_i

The pooled incidence rate ratio is estimated as a pooled odds ratio from the following formula.

$$OR_{\text{MH}} = \frac{\displaystyle\sum_i \frac{a_i d_i}{T_i}}{\displaystyle\sum_i \frac{b_i c_i}{T_i}} \tag{8–6}$$

The data in Table 8–6 are from a case-control study of congenital heart disease that examined the relation between spermicide use and Down

Table 8–6. Infants with congenital heart disease and Down syndrome and healthy controls, by maternal spermicide use before conception and maternal age at delivery*

| | *Maternal Age (years), Spermicide Use* | | | | | |
| | <35 | | | ≥35 | | |
	Yes	No	Total	Yes	No	Total
Cases	3	9	12	1	3	4
Controls	104	1059	1163	5	86	91
Total	107	1068	1175	6	89	95
Odds ratio		3.39			5.73	

*Data from Rothman.[6]

syndrome among the subset of cases that had both congenital heart disease and Down syndrome. The total congenital heart disease case series comprised more than 300 subjects, but the Down syndrome case series was a small subset of the original series that was of interest with regard to the specific issue of a possible relation with spermicide use. For the crude data, combining the above strata into a single table, the odds ratio is 3.50. Applying formula 8–6 gives us an estimate of the effect of spermicide use unconfounded by age.

$$OR_{MH} = \frac{\dfrac{3 \cdot 1059}{1175} + \dfrac{1 \cdot 86}{95}}{\dfrac{104 \cdot 9}{1175} + \dfrac{5 \cdot 3}{95}} = \frac{2.704 + 0.905}{0.797 + 0.158} = 3.78$$

This result is slightly larger than the crude estimate of 3.50, indicating that there was modest confounding by maternal age. We can obtain a confidence interval for the pooled estimate from the last variance formula in Table 8–4.

$$G_1 = 2.704 \qquad G_2 = 0.905$$
$$H_1 = 0.797 \qquad H_2 = 0.158$$
$$P_1 = 0.904 \qquad P_2 = 0.916$$
$$Q_1 = 0.096 \qquad Q_2 = 0.084$$

$Var[\ln(OR_{MH})]$

$$= \frac{2.704 \cdot 0.904 + 0.905 \cdot 0.916}{2(2.704 + 0.905)^2}$$

$$+ \frac{(2.704 \cdot 0.096 + 0.797 \cdot 0.904) + (0.905 \cdot 0.084 + 0.158 \cdot 0.916)}{2(2.704 + 0.905) \cdot (0.797 + 0.158)}$$

$$+ \frac{0.797 \cdot 0.096 + 0.158 \cdot 0.084}{2(0.797 + 0.158)^2}$$

$$= 0.126 + 0.174 + 0.049 = 0.349$$

The corresponding standard error is $0.349^{\frac{1}{2}} = 0.591$. The 90% confidence interval for the pooled odds ratio is calculated as follows:

$$OR_L = e^{\ln(3.78) - 1.645 \cdot 0.591} = 1.43$$

$$OR_U = e^{\ln(3.78) + 1.645 \cdot 0.591} = 10.0$$

Standardization

Standardization is a method of combining category-specific rates into a single summary value by taking a weighted average of them. It weights the category-specific rates using weights that come from a *standard* population. The weights, in fact, define the standard. Suppose one is standardizing a set of age-specific rates to conform to a specific age standard. One might decide to use the U.S. population in the year 2000 as the standard. That choice means that the weights used to average the age-specific rates reflect the distribution of the U.S. population in the year 2000. Standardization is thus a process of weighting the rates in two or more categories by a specified set of weights.

Suppose we have a rate of $10/1000 \text{ yr}^{-1}$ for males and a rate of $5/1000 \text{ yr}^{-1}$ for females. We can standardize these sex-specific rates to any standard that we wish. A reasonable standard might be one that weights males and females equally. We would then obtain a weighted average of the two rates that would equal $7.5/1000 \text{ yr}^{-1}$. Suppose the rates reflected the disease experience of nurses, 95% of whom are female. In that case, we might wish to use as a standard a weight of 5% for males and 95% for females. The standardized rate would then be as follows:

$$0.05 \times 10/1000 \text{ yr}^{-1} + 0.95 \times 5/1000 \text{ yr}^{-1} = 5.25/1000 \text{ yr}^{-1}$$

If all categories had similar rates, the choice of weights would matter little. Suppose that males and females had the same rate, $8.0/1000 \text{ yr}^{-1}$. Then the standardized rate, after standardizing for sex, would have to be $8.0/1000 \text{ yr}^{-1}$ because the standardization would involve taking a weighted average of two values, both of which were $8.0/1000 \text{ yr}^{-1}$. In such a situation, the choice of weights is not important. When rates do vary over categories, however, the choice of weights, which is to say the choice of a standard, can greatly affect the overall summary result. If the standard couples large weights with categories that have high rates, the standardized rate will be high, whereas if it assigns large weights to categories with low rates, the standardized rate will be low. Some epidemiologists prefer not to derive a summary measure when the value of the summary is so dependent on the choice of weights. On the other hand, it may be convenient or even necessary to obtain a single summary value, in which case a standardized rate provides at least some information about how the category-specific information was weighted, by disclosing which standard was used.

Although one can standardize a single set of rates, the main reason to standardize is to facilitate comparisons; therefore, there are usually two or more sets of rates that are standardized. If we wish to compare rates for exposed and unexposed people, we would standardize both groups to the same standard. The standardized comparison is akin to pooling. Both standardization and pooling involve comparing a weighted average of the stratum-specific results. With pooling, the weights for each stratum are buried within the Mantel-Haenszel formulas and, thus, are not immediately obvious. The built-in weights reflect the information content of the stratum-specific data. These Mantel-Haenszel weights are large for strata that have more information and small for strata that have less information. Because the weighting reflects the amount of information in each stratum, the result of pooling is an overall estimate that is optimal from the point of view of statistical efficiency. Standardization also assigns a weight to each stratum and involves taking a weighted average of the results across the strata. Unlike pooling, however, in standardization the weights may have nothing to do with the amount of data in each stratum. Thus, in pooling, the weights come from the data themselves, whereas in standardization, the weights can come from outside the data and simply reflect the distribution of the standard, which may correspond to a specific population or be chosen arbitrarily.

Standardization also differs from pooling in that pooling assumes that the effect is the same in all strata (often called the *assumption of uniformity of effect*). This assumption is the premise from which the formulas for pooling are derived. As explained earlier, even when the assumption of uniformity of effect is wrong, pooling may still be reasonable. We do not necessarily expect that the effect is strictly uniform across strata when we make the assumption of uniformity; rather, it is an assumption of convenience. We may be willing to tolerate substantial variation in the effect across strata as a price for the convenience and efficiency of pooling, as long as we are comfortable with the idea that the actual relation of the effect to the stratification variable is not strikingly different for different strata. When the effect is strikingly different for different strata, however, we can still use standardization to obtain a summary estimate of the effect across strata, because standardization has no requirement that the effect be uniform across strata.

Although standardization is preferable to pooling when an effect apparently varies across strata, standardization may be desirable even

Crude rates and standardized rates

A crude rate may be thought of as a weighted average of category-specific rates, in which the weights correspond to the actual distribution of the population. Consider age for the purpose of discussion. Every population can be divided into age categories. The age-specific rates in a population can be averaged to obtain an overall rate. If the averaging uses weights that reflect the amount of the population (or person-time) that actually falls into each age category, the weighted average that results is the crude rate. Algebraically, if each age-specific rate is denoted as A_i/PT_i, where A_i is the number of cases in age category i (ranging from 1 to K) and PT_i is the number of person-time units in that category, the crude rate is as follows:

$$\frac{PT_1\dfrac{A_1}{PT_1} + PT_2\dfrac{A_2}{PT_2} + \ldots + PT_K\dfrac{A_K}{PT_K}}{PT_1 + PT_2 + \ldots + PT_K} = \frac{\sum A_i}{\sum PT_i} = \frac{A}{PT}$$

A is the total number of cases in the population and PT is the total person-time. The crude rate is thus a weighted average of the age-specific rates, where the weights are the same as the denominators for the rates: $PT_1, PT_2, \ldots PT_K$. These are the *natural* weights, or *latent* weights, for the population. If we now change the weights from the denominator values of the rates to an outside set of weights, drawn from a standard, the resulting standardized rate can be viewed as the value that the crude rate would have been if the population age structure were changed from what it actually is to that of the standard, and the same age-specific rates applied. Thus, a standardized rate is a hypothetical crude rate that would apply if the age structure were that of the standard instead of what it happens to be.

when pooling is a reasonable alternative, simply because standardization uses a defined set of weights to combine results across strata. This characteristic of standardization provides for better comparability of stratified results from one study to another or within a study.

Consider the data on clozapine use and mortality in Table 8–5. We obtained a pooled estimate of the mortality rate difference, using the Mantel-Haenszel approach, of -720×10^{-5} yr^{-1}. Suppose we chose instead to standardize the rates for age over the two age categories. What age standard might we use? Let us standardize to the age distribution of current clozapine use in the study, since that is the age distribution of those who use the drug. There were a total of 68,204 person-years of current clozapine use, of which 62,119 (91.1%) were in the younger

---

What is an SMR?

When the standardized rate ratio is calculated using the exposed group as the standard, the result is usually referred to as a *standardized mortality, or morbidity, ratio* (SMR). The standardized rate ratio for clozapine that is calculated using the age distribution of current users as the age standard is an example of an SMR. An SMR can be expressed as the ratio of the total number of deaths in the exposed group, 363 in the clozapine example, divided by the number expected in the exposed group if the rates among the unexposed prevailed within each of the age categories. Thus, for the 10–54 age group, if the rate among past users of 704.2/100,000 yr^{-1} had prevailed among the 62,119 person-years experienced by current users, there would have been 437.4 deaths expected in that age category. Similar calculations give 343.6 deaths expected in the 55–94 age category. The figure for total expected deaths is 437.4 + 343.6 = 781.0. The SMR is the ratio of observed to expected deaths, which is 363/781.0 = 0.47. This result is algebraically identical to standardization based on taking a weighted average of the age-specific rates and taking the age distribution of current users as the standard.

The SMR is sometimes claimed to result from a method of standardization called indirect standardization, as opposed to direct standardization. That is a misnomer, however, as there is nothing indirect about indirect standardization. Indeed, the only feature that distinguishes it from supposedly direct standardization is that for an SMR the standard is always the exposed group. The calculations for any rate standardization, direct or indirect, are basically the same.

---

age category. To standardize the death rate for past users to this standard, we take a weighted average of past use as follows.

$$0.911 \times 704.2/100,000 \ yr^{-1} + 0.089 \times 5647/100,000 \ yr^{-1} = 1144/100,000 \ yr^{-1}$$

The standardized rate for current users, standardized to their age distribution, is the same as the crude rate for current users, which is 532.2/100,000 yr^{-1}. The *standardized rate difference* is the difference between the standardized rates for current and past users, which is (532.2 − 1144)/100,000 yr^{-1} = −612/100,000 yr^{-1}, slightly smaller in absolute value than the −720/100,000 yr^{-1} obtained from the pooled analysis. Analogously, we can obtain the *standardized rate ratio* by dividing the rate among current users by that among past users, giving 532.2/1144 = 0.47, essentially identical to the result obtained through pooling. The stratum-specific rate ratios did not vary much, so any weighting, whether pooled or standardized, will produce a result close to this value.

Both pooling and standardization can be used to control confounding.

Because they are different approaches and can give different results, it is fair to ask why we would want to use one rather than the other. Both involve taking weighted averages of the stratum-specific results. The difference is where the weights come from. In pooling, the data determine the weights, which are derived mathematically to give statistically optimal results. This method gives precise results (that is, relatively narrow confidence intervals), but the weights are statistical constructs that come out of the data and cannot easily be specified. Standardization, unlike pooling, may involve weights that are inefficient if large weights are assigned to strata with little data and vice versa. On the other hand, the weights are explicit. Ideally, the weights used in standardization should be presented along with the results. Making the weights used in standardization explicit facilitates comparison with other data. Thus, standardization may be less efficient, but it may provide for better comparability. For a more detailed discussion of standardization, including appropriate confidence interval formulas for standardized results, see Rothman and Greenland.[7]

In a stratified analysis, another option that is always open is to stratify the data and to present the results without aggregating the stratum-specific information over the strata. Stratification is highly useful even if it does not progress beyond examining the stratum-specific findings. This approach to presenting the data is especially attractive when the effect measure of interest appears to change considerably across the strata. In such a situation, a single summary estimate is less attractive an option than it would be in a situation in which the effect measure is nearly constant across strata.

Calculation of p Values for Stratified Data

Earlier, we gave the reasons why estimation is preferable to statistical significance testing. Nevertheless, for completeness, we give here the formulas for calculating p values from stratified data. These are straightforward extensions of the formulas presented in Chapter 7 for crude data.

For risk, prevalence, or case-control data, all of which consist of a set of 2×2 tables, the χ formula is as follows.

$$\chi = \frac{\sum_i a_i - \sum_i \frac{N_{1i}M_{1i}}{T_i}}{\sqrt{\sum_i \frac{N_{1i}N_{0i}M_{1i}M_{0i}}{T_i^2(T_i - 1)}}}$$

Applying this formula to the case-control data in Table 8–6 gives the following χ statistic.

$$\chi = \frac{(3 + 1) - \left(\dfrac{12 \cdot 107}{1175} + \dfrac{4 \cdot 6}{95} \right)}{\sqrt{\dfrac{107 \cdot 1068 \cdot 12 \cdot 1163}{1175^2 \cdot 1174} + \dfrac{6 \cdot 89 \cdot 4 \cdot 91}{95^2 \cdot 94}}} = 2.41$$

This result translates to a p value of 0.016 (see Appendix). For rate data, the corresponding formula is as follows.

$$\chi = \frac{\displaystyle\sum_i a_i - \sum_i \frac{PT_{1i}M_i}{T_i}}{\sqrt{\displaystyle\sum_i M_i \frac{PT_{1i}PT_{0i}}{T_i^2}}}$$

Applying this formula to the data in Table 8–5, we obtain the following.

$$\chi = \frac{(196 + 167) - \left(\dfrac{62,119 \cdot 307}{77,882} + \dfrac{6085 \cdot 324}{8865} \right)}{\sqrt{\dfrac{307 \cdot 62,119 \cdot 15,763}{77,882^2} + \dfrac{324 \cdot 6085 \cdot 2780}{8865^2}}} = -9.55$$

This result is too large, in absolute value, for the Appendix, implying an extremely small p value.

Measuring Confounding

The control of confounding and assessment of confounding are closely intertwined. It might seem reasonable to assess how much confounding a given variable produces in a body of data before we control for that confounding. The assessment might indicate, for example, that there is not enough confounding to present a problem, and we may therefore ignore that variable in the analysis. It is possible to predict the amount of confounding from the general characteristics of confounding variables, that is, the associations of a confounder with both exposure and disease. To measure confounding directly, however, requires that we control it: the procedure is to remove the confounding from the data and then see how much has been removed.

As an example of the measurement of confounding, let us return to the data in Tables 1–1 and 1–2. In Table 1–1, we have risks of death over a 20-year period of 0.24 among smokers and 0.31 among nonsmokers. The crude risk ratio is $0.24/0.31 = 0.76$, indicating a risk among smokers that is 24% lower than that among nonsmokers. As was indicated both in Chapter 1 and earlier in this chapter, this apparent protective effect of smoking on the risk of death is confounded by age, which can be seen from the data in Table 1–2. The age confounding can be removed by applying formula 8–2, which gives a result of 1.21. This value indicates a risk of death among smokers that is 21% greater than that of nonsmokers. The discrepancy between the crude risk ratio of 0.76 and the unconfounded risk ratio of 1.21 is a direct measure of age confounding. Were these two values equal, there would be no indication of confounding in the data. To the extent that they differ, it indicates the presence of age confounding. The age confounding is strong enough, in this instance, to have reversed the apparent effect of smoking, making it appear that smoking is related to a reduced risk of death in the crude data. This biased result occurs because smokers tend to be younger than nonsmokers, so the crude comparison between smokers and non-smokers is to some extent a comparison of younger women with older women, mixing the smoking effect with an age effect that negates it. By stratifying, the age confounding can be removed, revealing the adverse effect of smoking. The direct measure of this confounding effect is a comparison of the pooled estimate of the risk ratio with the crude estimate of the risk ratio.

A common mistake is to use statistical significance tests to evaluate the presence or absence of confounding. This mistaken approach to the evaluation of confounding applies a significance test to the association between a confounder and the exposure or the disease. The amount of confounding, however, is a result of the strength of the associations between the confounder and both exposure and disease. Confounding does not depend on the statistical significance of these associations. Furthermore, a significance test evaluates only one of the two component relations that give rise to confounding. Perhaps the most common situation in which this mistaken approach to evaluating confounding is applied is the analysis of randomized trials, when "baseline" characteristics are compared for the randomized groups. Baseline comparisons are useful, but often they are conducted with the sole aim of checking for statistically significant differences in any of the baseline variables, as a means of detecting confounding. A better way to evaluate confounding, in a trial as in any study, would be to control for the potential confounder and determine whether the unconfounded result differs from the crude, potentially confounded result.

Stratification by Two or More Variables

For convenience of presentation, the examples in this chapter have used few strata with only one stratification variable. Nevertheless, stratified analysis can be conducted with two or more stratification variables. Suppose that you wish to control confounding by sex and age simultaneously, with five age categories. The combination of age and sex categories will produce 10 strata. All of the methods discussed in this chapter can be applied without any modification to a stratified analysis with two or more stratification variables. The only real difficulty with such analyses is that with several variables to control the number of strata increases quickly and can stretch the data too far. Thus, to control five different variables with three categories each in a stratified analysis would require $3 \times 3 \times 3 \times 3 \times 3 = 243$ strata. With so many strata, many of them would contain few observations and end up contributing little information to the data summary. When the numbers within strata become very small, and in particular when zeroes become frequent in the tables, some tables may not contribute any information to the summary measures and some of the study information is effectively lost. As a result, the analysis as a whole becomes less precise. Thus, stratified analysis is not a practical method to control for many confounding factors at once. Fortunately, it is rare to have substantial confounding by many variables at once.

The Importance of Stratification

The formulas in this chapter may look imposing, but they can be applied readily with a hand calculator or a spreadsheet or even a pencil and paper. Consequently, the methods described here to control confounding are widely accessible without heavy reliance on technology. These are not the only methods available to control confounding. In Chapter 10, we discuss multivariable modeling to control confounding. Multivariable modeling requires computer hardware and software but offers the possibility of convenient methods to control confounding not merely for a single variable but simultaneously for a set of variables. The allure of these multivariable methods is nearly irresistible. Nevertheless, stratified analysis is preferable and should always be the method of choice to control confounding. This is not to say that multivariable modeling should be ignored: it does have its uses. Nevertheless, stratification is the preferred approach, at least as the initial approach to data analysis. Following are the main advantages of stratification over multivariable analysis.

1. With stratified analysis, the investigator can visualize the distribution of subjects by exposure, disease, and the potential confounder. Strange features in the distributions become immediately apparent. These distributions are obscure when conducting multivariable modeling.
2. Not only the investigator but also the consumer of the research will be able to visualize the distributions. Indeed, from detailed

tables of stratified data, a reader will be able to check the calculations or conduct his or her own pooled or standardized analysis.
3. Fewer assumptions are needed for a stratified analysis, reducing
the possibility of obtaining a biased result.

It should be standard practice to examine the data by categories of the
primary potential confounding factors, that is, to conduct a stratified
analysis. It is rare that a multivariable analysis will change the interpretation produced by a stratified analysis. The stratified analysis will
keep both the researcher and the reader better informed about the nature of the data. Even when it is reasonable to conduct a multivariable
analysis, it should be undertaken only after the researcher has conducted a stratified analysis and, thus, has a good appreciation for the
confounding in the data, or lack of it, by the main study variables.

Questions

1. In Table 8–3, the crude value of the risk ratio is 1.44, which is between
the values for the risk ratio in the two age strata. Could the crude risk
ratio have been outside the range of the stratum-specific values, or
must it always fall within the range of the stratum-specific values?
Why or why not?
2. The pooled estimate for the risk ratio from Table 8–3 was 1.33, also
within the range of the stratum-specific values. Does the pooled estimate always fall within the range of the stratum-specific estimates of
the risk ratio? Why or why not?
3. If you were comparing the effect of exposure at several levels and
needed to control confounding, would you prefer to compare a pooled
estimate of the effect at each level or a standardized estimate of the
effect at each level? Why?
4. Prove that an SMR is "directly" standardized to the distribution of the
exposed group; that is, prove that an SMR is the ratio of two standardized rates that are both standardized to the distribution of the
exposed group.
5. Suppose that an investigator conducting a randomized trial of an old
and a new treatment examines baseline characteristics of the subjects
(such as age, sex, or stage of disease) that might be confounding factors and finds that the two groups are different with respect to several
characteristics. Why is it unimportant whether these differences are
"statistically significant"?
6. Suppose one of the differences in question 5 is statistically significant. A
significance test is a test of the null hypothesis, which is a hypothesis
that chance alone can account for the observed difference. What is the
explanation for baseline differences in a randomized trial? What implication does that explanation have for dealing with these differences?

7. The larger a randomized trial, the less the possibility for confounding. Why? Explain why the size of a study does not affect confounding in nonexperimental studies.
8. Imagine a stratum of a case-control study in which all subjects were unexposed. What is the mathematical contribution of that stratum to the estimate of the pooled odds ratio (formula 8–6)? What is the mathematical contribution of that stratum to the variance of the pooled odds ratio (bottom formula in Table 8–4)?

References

1. Rothman KJ, Monson RR: Survival in trigeminal neuralgia. *J Chron Dis* 1973;26:303–309.
2. Mantel N, Haenszel WH Statistical aspects of the analysis of data from retrospective studies of disease. *J. Natl. Cancer Inst.* 1959;22:719–748.
3. University Group Diabetes Program. A study of the effects of hypoglycemic agents on vascular complications in patients with adult onset diabetes. *Diabetes* 1970;19(Suppl. 2):747–830.
4. Rothman KJ, Greenland S: *Modern Epidemiology*, Second Edition. Lippincott-Raven, Philadelphia, 1998, pp 275–279.
5. Walker AM, Lanza LL, Arellano F, Rothman KJ: Mortality in current and former users of clozapine. *Epidemiology* 1997;8:671–677.
6. Rothman KJ: Spermicide use and Down syndrome. *Am J Public Health.* 1982;72:399–401.
7. Rothman KJ, Greenland S: *Modern Epidemiology*, Second Edition. Lippincott-Raven, Philadelphia, 1998, pp 260–265.

9

Measuring Interactions

The nature of causal mechanisms is complicated enough that we expect some causes to have an effect only under certain conditions. This principle is illustrated by the observation that even among the heaviest of cigarette smokers, only 1 in 10 will develop lung cancer during their lives. If we accept the proposition that cigarette smoking causes lung cancer, this observation implies that the complementary causes that act together with cigarette smoking to cause lung cancer play their causal role in only 10% of heavy smokers. These complementary causes interact biologically with cigarette smoke. Some form of causal interaction occurs in every case of every disease, so there is good reason for epidemiologists to be interested in interaction. Unfortunately, there is substantial confusion surrounding the evaluation of interaction, much of which stems from the fact that the term is used differently in statistics and in epidemiology.

Knowledge about causal interactions is not just of academic interest; it has important public-health implications. By identifying groups or settings in which interaction occurs, preventive actions can be more effective. Following are some examples of how knowledge of causal interactions affects public health: (1) Influenza can lead to serious complications, but those at highest risk of complications are youngsters, the elderly, and people with heart and lung disorders. These groups can be targeted for influenza vaccination. (2) People who do get influenza are sometimes treated with aspirin. A rare but potentially deadly consequence of aspirin therapy is Reye's syndrome, which can also occur without aspirin use but is more likely to occur among youngsters who take aspirin for a viral illness. Rather than deter everyone from using aspirin, which is a useful drug with many indications in adults, epidemiologic knowledge of the interaction between aspirin and age has enabled preventive efforts to focus on discouraging aspirin use only in children. (3) One of the best-known efforts based on a causal interaction is the public-health campaign against drunk driving. Both driving and alcohol consumption are risk factors for injury, but their combination is a much more potent cause of injury than either alone.

Effect-Measure Modification

In statistics, the term "interaction" is used to refer to departure from the underlying form of a statistical model. Because there are various statistical models, interaction does not have a consistent, universal meaning. This ambiguity has a counterpart in epidemiology, in the term *effect-measure modification*, which refers to the common situation in which a measure of effect changes over values of some other variable. Suppose that we are measuring the effect of an exposure and that the other variable is age. Consider the age-incidence curves in Figure 9–1. The rate of disease rises linearly with age among those who are unexposed. If it rose linearly with the same slope among those who are exposed, as depicted by the other solid line in Figure 9–1, the difference between incidence rates among the exposed and unexposed would be constant with age. In that case, we would say that age does not modify the rate difference measure of effect. Looking at the same two curves, however, we can see that the rate ratio measure of effect does change with age: the ratio of the incidence rate among the exposed to that among the unexposed is large at young ages and small at older ages, despite the constant rate difference. The reason that the ratio declines with age is the steady rise in the rate among the unexposed with age.

Figure 9–1 also illustrates an alternative situation, in which the rate

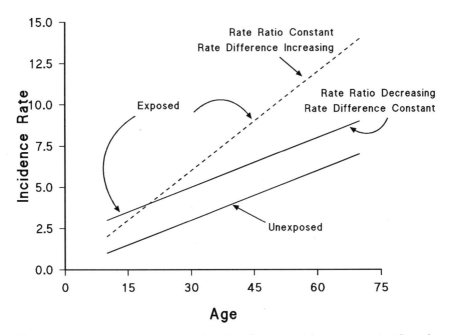

Figure 9–1. Age-incidence curves showing disease incidence increasing linearly with age for unexposed and two possible linear relations over age for exposed.

among the exposed increases linearly with age so that the ratio of the rate among the exposed to that among the unexposed remains constant over age; this alternative is depicted by the dashed line. In this alternative situation, we would say that because the rate ratio is constant over age, age does not modify the rate ratio effect measure. The rate difference measure, however, increases with age, as is evident from the increasing distance between the dashed line for exposed and the line for unexposed as age increases. From these examples it is easy to see that even in the unusual situation in which one of the effect measures is not modified by age, the other is likely to be modified. Thus, we typically cannot make a blanket statement about the presence or absence of effect-measure modification because the answer depends on which effect measure is under discussion.

Effect modification versus effect-measure modification

Epidemiologists often use the term *effect modification* to mean what is described here as effect-measure modification. The addition of the word *measure* to the phrase is intended to emphasize the dependence of this phenomenon on the choice of the effect measure and its consequent ambiguity. One cannot speak in general terms about the presence or absence of effect modification, any more than one can speak in general terms about the presence or absence of clouds in the sky, without being more specific as to the details. For clouds in the sky, the details would include the geographic area, the time, and perhaps what is meant by a cloud. In the case of effect-measure modification, the details are in the choice of effect measure.

Consider the hypothetical data in Table 9–1 on risk of lung cancer according to two environmental exposures, cigarette smoke and asbestos. What can we say about how exposure to smoking modifies the effect of asbestos? Suppose that we measure the risk difference. Among non-smokers, the risk difference for the effect of asbestos is $5 - 1 = 4$ cases per 100,000. Among smokers, the risk difference is $50 - 10 = 40$ cases per 100,000, 10 times as great. On this basis, we would say that smoking is an effect modifier of the risk difference measuring the effect of asbestos. If we looked at the risk ratio instead, however, we would find that the risk ratio measuring an effect of asbestos is 5 among non-smokers and 5 among smokers. Therefore, smoking does not modify the risk ratio of the asbestos effect. Is smoking an effect-measure modifier of the asbestos effect? It is and it is not, depending on which effect measure that we use. This example, like the previous one, illustrates the ambiguity of the concept of effect-measure modification. The example could be turned around: one could ask whether asbestos modifies the effect of

Table 9–1. Hypothetical 1-year risk of lung cancer according to exposure to cigarette smoke and to asbestos (cases per 100,000)

	No Asbestos Exposure	Asbestos Exposure
Nonsmokers	1	5
Smokers	10	50

smoking. The pattern is symmetrical, and the answer is the same: the risk difference of the smoking effect is modified by asbestos exposure, but the risk ratio is not.

The ambiguity of the concept of effect-measure modification corresponds directly to the ambiguity of the concept of statistical interaction. Statistical models used in epidemiology are discussed in Chapter 10. If a statistical model is based on additivity of effects, such as an ordinary linear regression model, the data in Table 9–1 would indicate the presence of statistical interaction, because the separate effects of smoking and asbestos are not additive when both are present. If a statistical model is based on the multiplication of relative effects, as is the case for many popular statistical models used in epidemiologic applications (logistic regression is one example), the data in Table 9–1 would indicate no statistical interaction because the relative effects of smoking and asbestos are multiplicative: the risk ratio of smoking alone, 10, multiplied by the risk ratio of asbestos alone, 5, gives the risk ratio of 50 for those with smoking and asbestos exposure compared with those who have neither.

These examples illustrate the ambiguity of both effect-measure modification and statistical interaction. Both depend on an arbitrary choice of measure or of scale. Statistical interaction, being ambiguous, cannot correspond to the concept of biologic interaction among component causes. Biologic interaction refers to a mechanistic interaction that either exists or does not exist. It is not a feature that can be turned off or on by an arbitrary choice of an effect measure or statistical model. Statistical interaction, therefore, should not be confused with biologic interaction. Unfortunately, when statistical interaction is discussed, it is usually described as simply "interaction," and is thus often confused with biologic interaction. Often, the only way to distinguish one from the other is by a careful reading of what is being reported or described. Here, we use the terms *biologic interaction* and *statistical interaction* to keep these concepts separate.

As stated earlier, biologic interaction between two causes occurs whenever the effect of one is dependent on the presence of the other. For example, being exposed to someone with an active measles infection is a causal risk factor for getting measles, but the effect of the exposure depends on another risk factor, lack of immunity. Someone who has been vaccinated or has already had measles will not experience any effect

---

Pooling and a multiplicative relation

In a stratified analysis using pooling, a necessary assumption is that the effect measure is constant over strata. If the effect measure is the risk ratio or the rate ratio, then pooling requires the assumption that the risk ratio or rate ratio is constant over strata. This assumption amounts to an assumption of a multiplicative relation between the exposure and the stratification variable. In Table 9–1, suppose that asbestos is the exposure and the data are stratified by smoking. Within the stratum of nonsmokers, the risk ratio for asbestos is 5/1 or 5. Within the stratum of smokers, the risk ratio for asbestos is 50/10 or 5. Thus, the risk ratio for asbestos is 5 within each stratum of smoking. The relation is symmetrical: if we consider smoking to be the exposure and asbestos to be the stratification variable, we find that the risk ratio for smoking is 10 within each stratum of asbestos. Thus, a uniform risk ratio across strata is equivalent to a multiplicative relation between exposure and the stratification variable. Because a multiplicative relation is evidence of a biologic interaction, pooling to estimate a uniform risk ratio requires us to assume that there is a biologic interaction between the exposure and the stratification variable. This implicit assumption is not necessarily a problem with pooling, but it is a feature of stratified analysis worth keeping in mind.

---

from being exposed to someone with an active measles infection. The effect is limited to people who lack immunity. Lack of immunity is sometimes referred to as *susceptibility,* a term that refers to the condition of having one of two interacting causes already and therefore being susceptible to the effect of the other. (Other terms commonly used to describe aspects of biologic interaction include *predisposition, promotion, predisposing factor,* and *cofactor.*) Another example of biologic interaction is the development of melanoma among those with high levels of exposure to ultraviolet light who also have fair skin. Dark skin protects against the adverse effects of ultraviolet light exposure, whereas those with fair skin experience a much greater risk from ultraviolet light exposure. Many environmental causes of disease interact with genetic predisposing factors. People who carry the predisposing gene constitute a group that has high susceptibility to the environmental factors. Thus, people who carry a gene that codes for faulty receptor sites for low-density lipoprotein (or "bad" cholesterol) will experience a greater risk from a diet high in saturated fat than those who do not carry that gene. For these genetically predisposed people, the effect of the dietary exposure to saturated fat interacts with the presence of the gene to cause disease.

A Definition of Biologic Interaction

How can we derive an unambiguous definition of biologic interaction? We have already described what we mean by interaction between causes in terms of the sufficient/component cause model: the coparticipation in a causal mechanism of two or more component causes. Interaction between causes A and B in a given instance corresponds to the occurrence of a case of disease in which both A and B played a causal role. It means that both A and B were part of the causal mechanism for that case, or in terms of the model, both A and B were parts of the same causal pie. Factors A and B can both be causes of the same disease without interacting, but for that to happen, they would have to be causes of different cases. It is possible that A plays a role in causal mechanisms in which B does not and vice versa. Under those circumstances, some cases would occur from causal mechanisms involving A and others from causal mechanisms involving B; both factors would act independently as causes of the disease.

With regard to the interaction of factors A and B, there are four possible classes of causal mechanism into which all causal mechanisms of the disease fall. These classes are diagramed in Figure 9–2.

The first class in Figure 9–2 comprises those mechanisms in which A and B interact in producing the disease. The piece of the causal pie labeled U refers to the unidentified complementary component causes that also interact with A and B to produce disease. Because U could represent many different combinations of component causes that act in concert with A and B in the same mechanism, we refer to these as a set, or class, of causal mechanisms. Within this class of mechanisms, every causal mechanism includes among the component causes both A and B. If either A or B were absent in a given person, that person could not get disease through any mechanism in this class. Thus, cases that occur through these mechanisms would not have occurred if either A or B had not been present. We can therefore say that these cases are dependent on the joint presence of A and B.

The second and third classes of mechanisms in Figure 9–2 represent causal mechanisms in which either A or B plays a causal role but the other does not. Again, U refers to unidentified complementary compo-

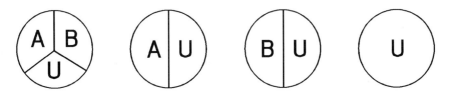

Figure 9–2. Four classes of causal mechanism involving component causes A and B.

nent causes other than A or B and could represent various combinations of complementary causes, explaining why each pie is an entire class of mechanism. The fourth class of mechanisms, often referred to as the background occurrence, refers to causal mechanisms that produce disease without either A or B playing any causal role. The solitary U in that pie represents all combinations of causal components that can cause the disease, with the proviso that these combinations do not include A or B. The background occurrence represents disease mechanisms that are independent of the causal action of A or B.

One way to measure the interaction between A and B would be to measure the risk of developing disease caused by mechanisms in which both A and B played a role. That is, we might measure the risk of disease caused by mechanisms in the first class in Figure 9–2. There is no way by direct observation alone that we can tell which class of causal mechanism is involved in the causation of individual cases. Even if a person were exposed to both A and B and developed the disease, it is possible that the disease could have been caused by a causal mechanism in any of the classes in Figure 9–2 and that one or both of the exposures A and B was just an incidental characteristic that did not play a causal role for that case of disease. We can, however, indirectly estimate the risk of becoming a case through mechanisms involving both A and B. We start by measuring risk among people exposed to both factors A and B. Cases of disease among people exposed to both A and B will include cases that occur from all four classes of mechanism in Figure 9–2. We narrow down to the first class of mechanism in Figure 9–2 by subtraction. For simplicity, we assume that all risks are low and we ignore competing risks.

Let us denote R_{AB} as the risk of disease among those with exposure to both A and B. As stated above, this risk comprises all four classes of mechanism in Figure 9–2. Let us now subtract the component of risk that corresponds to the risk of getting disease from mechanisms that include factor A but not B. We can estimate this component of the risk by measuring the disease risk among people exposed to A but not B. We will call this risk R_A. People exposed to A but not B cannot get disease from any causal mechanism that involves B. Therefore, the first and third classes of mechanism in Figure 9–2 do not occur among these people. These people can get disease through mechanisms that involve A but not B and from mechanisms that involve neither A nor B (the background). Thus, of the original four classes of causal mechanisms the expression $R_{AB} - R_A$ leaves the class of causal mechanisms involving interaction between A and B and the class of causal mechanisms involving factor B without factor A. (For this subtraction of risks to be valid, we have to assume that there was no confounding, which we must always assume when we use the risk or rate in one group to estimate what would happen in another group under counterfactual circumstances.)

Next, to eliminate the class of mechanism that involves B without A, we subtract the risk of disease among those with exposure B. This subtraction removes disease mechanisms that involve B without A, but it also subtracts disease mechanisms that involve neither B nor A (the background). As the background was already subtracted once when we subtracted R_A, if we subtract it a second time with R_B we need to add it back again. We then have the following equation.

$$\text{Interaction risk} = R_{AB} - R_A - R_B + R_U \qquad (9–1)$$

Expression 9–1 is a risk measure of the interaction between factors A and B in causing disease. Specifically, it is the risk of getting disease caused by mechanisms in which A and B interact. If this expression is 0, we say that there is no interaction between A and B, which means that A and B act only as causes in distinct causal mechanisms, rather than acting together in the same mechanism. By setting 9–1 equal to 0, which corresponds to no interaction, we can derive the expression that gives the relation of risks if A and B are biologically independent.

$$\text{Interaction risk} = 0 = R_{AB} - R_A - R_B + R_U$$

$$R_{AB} = R_A + R_B - R_U$$

$$(R_{AB} - R_U) = (R_A - R_U) + (R_B - R_U) \qquad (9–2)$$

Equation 9–2 expresses the relation between the risks under biologic independence. In words, this equation says that the risk difference between those with joint exposure to A and B compared with those who have neither exposure is equal to the sum of the risk differences for the effect of exposure to A in the absence of B and of exposure to B in the absence of A, both compared with the risk among those who lack exposure to both A and B (the background risk). In short, the risk differences are additive under independence.

Because equation 9–2 involves absolute risks, it appears to be useful only for cohort studies, in which risks can be measured. Is there an analogous expression for case-control studies, from which risk ratios can be estimated but risks and risk differences are not obtainable? To obtain an equivalent expression for risk ratios, we need only divide each term in equation 9–2 by the background risk, R_U.

$$(RR_{AB} - 1) = (RR_A - 1) + (RR_B - 1) \qquad (9–3)$$

In equation 9–3, RR_{AB} denotes the risk ratio for those exposed jointly to A and B compared with those exposed to neither (for whom the risk is R_U); RR_A denotes the risk ratio for those exposed to A but not B compared with R_U, and RR_B denotes the risk ratio for those exposed to B but not A compared with R_U. All of the risk ratios in equation 9–3 can be obtained from a case-control study that measures the effect of factors A and B.

Partitioning Risk Among Those with Joint Exposure

Equations 9–2 and 9–3 allow us to predict the risk or the risk ratio that would occur under biologic independence for those exposed jointly to two factors. In fact, these equations allow us to partition the observed risk of disease for those with exposure to A and B into four components that correspond to the four classes of causal mechanism depicted in Figure 9–2. As an illustration, let us partition the risk in Table 9–1 for those jointly exposed to cigarette smoke and asbestos into its four components. The value of the risk for those with joint exposure is 50 cases per 100,000. From Table 9–1, the risk among those who were nonsmokers and not exposed to asbestos is 1. The latter value is the background risk, or the background component of the partition of the risk among those with joint exposure. That means that for every 50 cases of lung cancer occurring among those who smoke and were exposed to asbestos, we would expect an average of 1 to occur from background causes that involve neither A nor B. How many cases would we expect from smoking acting in the absence of asbestos? The risk difference for smokers who are not exposed to asbestos is $10 - 1 = 9$ cases per 100,000. Thus, among every 50 cases who were smokers and exposed to asbestos, we would expect that 9 cases would occur from smoking through causal mechanisms that do not involve asbestos. Similarly, from the risk difference for asbestos alone, we would expect 4 cases to occur from mechanisms involving asbestos but not smoking. These three components add to $1 + 9 + 4 = 14$. We have so far accounted for 14 cases out of every 50 that occur among those with joint exposure. Under biologic independence, we would expect the risk among those who smoked and were exposed to asbestos to be 14; this is the value if there is no interaction. The excess above 14 corresponds to the effect of interaction between A and B. This excess is 36 cases out of 50. Thus, most of the risk among those with both exposures is attributable to interaction. Every 50 cases among those with both exposures can be partitioned into background (1 case), the effect of smoking alone (9 cases), the effect of asbestos alone (4 cases), and interaction between smoking and asbestos (36 cases). Thus, the data in Table 9–1 show considerable biologic interaction; quantitatively, we would say that 36/50, or 72%, of the cases occurring among those with joint exposure are attributable to causal mechanisms in which both factors play a causal role, which is to say that 72% of cases are attributable to biologic interaction.

As another example, let us consider the risk ratio data in Table 9–2, reporting on the interaction between oral contraceptives and hypertension in the causation of stroke.

Table 9–2. Risk ratio of stroke by exposure to oral contraceptives and presence or absence of hypertension*

Oral Contraceptive Use	No Hypertension	Hypertension
Nonusers	1.0	6.9
Users	3.1	13.6

*Data from Collaborative Group for The Study of Stroke in Young Women.[1]

These data come from a case-control study, but we can use the same approach as we used for the lung cancer data in Table 9–1 to evaluate interaction. The idea, once again, is to partition the effect measure for those with joint exposure into four parts: the background effect, the effect relating to each of the two exposures in the absence of the other, and the effect attributable to the biologic interaction. The risk ratio for those who are hypertensive and used oral contraceptives is 13.6. The background component is 1.0 out of 13.6 because the value of 1.0 for the risk ratio is by definition the value among those with neither exposure. What is the effect of oral contraceptives in the absence of hypertension? Among those without hypertension, oral-contraceptive users had a risk ratio of 3.1, which means that oral-contraceptive use increased the risk ratio from 1.0 to 3.1. The difference, 2.1, is the effect of oral contraceptives in the absence of hypertension. Similarly, we can see that the effect of hypertension in the absence of oral-contraceptive use is 6.9 − 1.0 = 5.9. That gives us three of the four components of the 13.6: 1.0 for the background, 2.1 for oral contraceptives alone, and 5.9 for hypertension alone. The remainder, 4.6, equals the part of the risk ratio that is attributable to the interaction between oral-contraceptive use and hypertension in the causation of stroke. As we did above, we can describe the amount of interaction by estimating the proportion of stroke cases, among women with hypertension who also use oral contraceptives, that is attributable to the interaction of these two causes. This proportion would be 4.6/13.6 = 34%. It would be zero, of course, if the two causes were biologically independent; the fact that about one-third of all cases are due to biologic interaction between the two causes indicates that the interaction is important.

The data in Table 9–2 provide an interesting contrast between the evaluation of biologic interaction and statistical interaction. A purely statistical approach to these case-control data would ordinarily fit a multiplicative model to the data because such models are typically used for the analysis of case-control data (see Chapter 10). Using a multiplicative model, we would find that there is statistical interaction in the data in Table 9–2, but that it goes in the opposite direction to the biologic interaction that we have just described. A multiplicative model would predict a value of the risk ratio among women who used oral contracep-

Assessing interaction with preventive factors

The approach to measuring interaction described in this chapter involves partitioning the cases that have simultaneous exposure to two factors into four subsets, according to the types of causal mechanism involved. The method assumes that both factors are causes, rather than preventives. When both factors are preventives or one is a cause and the other is a preventive, the assessment can be more complicated. It is possible to avoid the complication of preventive factors, however, if one chooses the high-risk category of both factors to be the exposed category. This technique changes a preventive factor into a causal factor by considering lack of the preventive to be the cause. For example, suppose that a vaccine prevents disease. One can say that being unvaccinated is a cause of disease. Similarly, if regular exercise reduces the risk of cardiovascular disease, we could just as well say that the absence of regular exercise increases the risk. By defining the exposure category so that each factor is viewed as a cause of disease, we can avoid the problem of dealing with preventive factors in assessing interaction.

tives and who were hypertensive based on the product of the individual risk ratios. Such a model predicts that the risk ratio for joint exposure is $3.1 \times 6.9 = 21.4$, whereas the observed risk ratio for the group with joint exposure was 13.6. Thus, evaluation of statistical interaction based on a multiplicative model indicates that those with joint exposure have a smaller effect than that predicted from the separate effects of the two causes. This conclusion is strikingly different from that which emerges from an evaluation of biologic interaction, as we have shown above. The evaluation of statistical interaction means only that the effect in those with joint exposure is less than multiplicative; it has no biologic implication. The data in this example demonstrate how misleading it can be to examine statistical interaction when the interest is in the biologic interaction between two causes. If multiplicative models are used as the baseline from which to measure (statistical) interaction, it will lead to an estimate of interaction that is smaller than an evaluation based on departures from additivity of risk differences. In the worst-case scenario, such as in this example of stroke, the two approaches can be so different that they point in opposite directions.

Why is it that biologic interaction should be evaluated as departures from additivity of effect? Perhaps the easiest way to understand the connection between additivity and biologic independence is to reflect on the derivation of equation 9–2, which establishes additivity as the definition of biologic independence. This derivation depends on the concept that we can partition all cases that occur among those with joint exposure into the four causal subsets depicted in Figure 9–2. Partitioning a collection into subsets is an operation that can be understood when dealing with an enumerated collection, but it does not make much sense if one were to invoke scale transformations. Multiplicative models typically involve logarithmic transformations. Once one takes the logarithm of the number of cases, however, partitioning no longer makes sense. The partitioning can be understood only on the original scale in which the cases are enumerated; therefore, the definition of biologic interaction is linked logically to the original scale. This linkage leads to a situation in which biologic independence results in additivity of risk differences. A more thorough discussion of this topic is given in Chapter 18 of *Modern Epidemiology*.[2]

Although multivariate modeling is not discussed until the next chapter, it is worth noting here that most of the multivariate models in com-

---

Independence is not a model

Some writers have pointed out that under certain circumstances we should expect to see variables have a multiplicative relation, and under other circumstances we might expect to see an additive relation. They have used this observation to argue in favor of flexibility for choosing different types of model in epidemiologic analysis. The argument is flawed, however, if it is used to suggest that we be flexible about which model to use as a starting point from which to measure interaction. The main problem is confusion between the goal of modeling, which is to find a succinct mathematical expression to explain the patterns in the data, and the goal of measuring biologic interaction, which requires that we know what the reference point is from which we measure the interaction. The reference point for measuring biologic interaction is additivity of risk differences; the derivation is given in the text. Taking this reference point as the definition of biologic independence is not the same as applying an additive model; in fact, it is not modeling at all. It may be that two causes have a multiplicative relation, as they do in Table 9–1. Nevertheless, even then, the amount of biologic interaction in the data is measured by taking the excess over additive effects. Doing so does not amount to application of an additive model, or of any model, but, rather, application of a specific definition of biologic independence. It is important to avoid confusion between modeling, on the one hand, and defining the relation specified by biologic independence, on the other hand. We can be flexible in modeling, but there is no room for arbitrariness when defining biologic independence. In short, evaluating interaction is not the same as choosing a statistical model.

mon use for epidemiologic data employ logarithmic transformations. As a result, attempting to evaluate interaction from these models using the conventional statistical approaches (the inclusion of "product terms" in the model) amounts to an evaluation of departures from a multiplicative model rather than departures from additivity. Thus, statistical evaluation of interaction using these models will not give an appropriate assessment of biologic interaction. It is possible, however, to use multivariate models to assess biologic interaction appropriately; in fact, it is straightforward. The method for doing so is given in the next chapter.

Questions

1. Explain why the mere observation that not every cigarette smoker gets lung cancer implies that cigarette smoking interacts with other factors in causing lung cancer.
2. From the data in Table 9–2, estimate the proportion of stroke cases among hypertensive women who use oral contraceptives that is attributable to the causal role of oral contraceptives.
3. In an analysis of the effect of oral contraceptives on stroke based on the data in Table 9–2, suppose that you were interested in the oral-contraceptive effect and wished only to control for possible confounding by hypertension using stratification. What would be the stratum-specific risk ratio estimates for oral-contraceptive use for the two strata of hypertension? In an ordinary stratified analysis, why is there a separate referent category in each stratum?
4. Show that if there is an excess over a multiplicative effect among those with joint exposure to two causes, there will also be an excess over an additive effect.
5. The investigators of the study described in Table 9–2 claimed that women who faced increased risk from one factor ought to avoid additional risk from another factor, regardless of whether the two factors interacted in the causation of the disease. Does this suggestion make sense? What would it imply about seat-belt use for women who take oral contraceptives?
6. List reasons why the study of biologic interaction is more difficult than the study of the effects of single factors.

References

1. Collaborative Group for the Study of Stroke in Young Women: Oral contraceptives and stroke in young women. *JAMA* 1975;231:718–722.
2. Rothman KJ, Greenland, S: *Modern Epidemiology,* 2nd ed, Concepts of Interaction. pp. 329–342. Philadelphia: Lippincott-Raven, 1998.

10

Using Regression Models in Epidemiologic Analysis

The straight line depicted in Figure 10–1 is an example of a simple mathematical model. It is a model because we use the mathematical equation for the straight line that is fitted to the data as a way of describing the relation between the two variables in the graph, cigarette smoking and laryngeal cancer mortality. We use models in epidemiology for various purposes. The two primary purposes are prediction and to control for confounding. Prediction models are used to estimate risk (or other epidemiologic measures) based on information from risk predictors. Thus, an equation can be used to estimate a person's risk of heart attack during a 10-year period based on information about the person's age, sex, family history, blood pressure, smoking history, weight, height, exercise habits, and medical history. Values for each of these predictors could be inserted into an equation that predicts the risk of heart attack from the combination of risk factors. The model must have terms in it for all of the risk factors listed.

In contrast to the goal of risk prediction for specific people, much epidemiologic research is aimed at learning about the causal role of specific factors for disease. In causal research, models are used to evaluate the causal role of one or more factors while simultaneously controlling for possible confounding effects of other factors. Because this use of multivariable models differs from the use of models to obtain estimates of risk for people, there are different considerations that apply to the construction of multivariable models for causal research. Unfortunately, many courses in statistics do not distinguish between the use of multivariable models for predicting individual estimates of risk and the use of such models for causal inference.

The data in Figure 10–1 illustrate a nearly perfect linear relation between the number of cigarettes smoked per day and the age-standardized mortality rate of laryngeal cancer. Seldom do epidemiologic data conform to such a striking linear pattern. The line drawn through the data points is a *regression line,* meaning that it estimates average values for

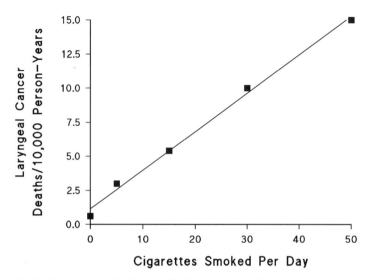

Figure 10–1. Age-standardized mortality from laryngeal cancer according to number of cigarettes smoked daily, derived from data of Kahn[1] (adapted from Rothman et al.[2] with permission of the *American Journal of Epidemiology*).

the variable on the vertical scale (Y) according to values of the variable on the horizontal scale (X). In this case, it is a *simple regression* because it can be described as a single straight line in the following form: $Y = a_0 + a_1X$. In this equation, a_0 is the intercept, which is the value of Y when X is 0; a_1 is the coefficient of X and describes the slope of the line, which is the number of units of change in Y for every unit change in X. In the figure, Y is the age-standardized mortality rate from laryngeal cancer; and X is the number of cigarettes smoked daily. The equation for the regression line in Figure 10–1 is $Y = 1.15 + 0.282X$. These values refer to deaths per 10,000 person-years. The intercept, 1.15, represents the number of deaths per 10,000 person-years that are estimated to occur in the absence of cigarette smoking. There is also a direct observation for the rate at the 0 level of smoking, which is 0.6 deaths per 10,000 person-years. The regression line estimates a slightly larger value, 1.15, than the value that was observed; this estimate is based on not just the 0 level for smoking but on all five data points. The regression line slope of 0.282 indicates that the number of deaths per 10,000 person-years is estimated to increase by 0.282 for every additional cigarette smoked daily.

Assuming that confounding and other biases have been properly addressed, the slope value of 0.282 quantifies the effect of cigarette smoking on death from laryngeal cancer. The regression line also allows us to estimate mortality rate ratios at different smoking levels. For example, from the regression line, we can estimate a mortality rate at 50 cigarettes daily (equivalent to 2.5 packs/day) of 15.2. Compared with the estimated rate among nonsmokers of 1.15, the rate ratio for smoking 2.5

packs daily is $15.2/1.15 = 13.3$. Put in these terms, we can readily see that the regression coefficient indicates a strong effect of smoking on laryngeal cancer mortality.

The General Linear Model

Models that incorporate terms for more than one factor at a time can be used as an alternative to stratification to achieve control of confounding. These models succeed in controlling confounding because when several risk factors are included, the effect of each is unconfounded by the others. Let us consider an extension of the simple linear model in Figure 10–1 to a third variable.

$$Y = a_0 + a_1X_1 + a_2X_2 \tag{10–1}$$

Equation 10–1 is also that of a straight line. The equation, like the one for the line in Figure 10–1, has one outcome variable (Y, also known as the *dependent* variable); but there are now two predictor, or *independent*, variables. Suppose that Y is the mortality rate from laryngeal cancer, as in Figure 10–1, and that X_1, as before, is the number of cigarettes smoked daily. The new variable, X_2, might be the number of grams of alcohol consumed daily (alcohol is also a risk factor for laryngeal cancer). With two independent variables and one dependent variable, the data points must now be visualized as being located within a three-dimensional space: two dimensions for the two independent variables and one dimension for the dependent variable. Imagine a room with the line where one wall meets the floor being the axis for X_1 and the line where the adjacent wall meets the floor being the axis for X_2. The line from floor to ceiling where these two walls meet would be the Y axis. Equation 10–1 is a straight line through the three-dimensional space of this room.

What is the advantage of adding the extra term to the model? Ordinarily, because cigarette smoking and alcohol consumption are correlated, we might expect that they would be mutually confounding risk factors for laryngeal cancer. A stratified analysis could remove that confounding, but the confounding can also be removed by fitting equation 10–1 to the data. In a model such as equation 10–1, which contains terms for two predictive factors, smoking (X_1) and alcohol (X_2), the coefficients for these terms, a_1 and a_2, respectively, provide estimates of the effects of cigarette smoking and alcohol drinking that are mutually unconfounded. Mathematically, there is no limit to the number of terms that can be included as independent variables in a model, although limitations of the data provide a practical limit. The general form of equation 10–1 is referred to as the *general linear model*.

Transforming the General Linear Model

The dependent variable in a regression model is not constrained mathematically to any specific range of values. In actual epidemiologic applications, however, the dependent variable might be constrained in various ways. For example, the dependent variable might be FEV_1 (forced expiratory volume in 1 second), a measure of lung function that cannot be negative. As another example, the dependent variable might be the occurrence of disease, which is measured as either no or yes and usually assigned a value of 0 or 1. It is common when using constrained outcome variables to use a transformation to avoid getting impossible values for the dependent variable. For example, the straight line in Figure 10–1 has an intercept of 1.15 deaths per 100,000 person-years. With some of the data points shifted only slightly, however, it would have been possible to have the line cross the Y axis at a value below 0, implying a negative mortality rate for nonsmokers. A negative mortality rate is impossible, of course, but there is nothing in the fitting of a straight line that confines the line to positive territory.

How could we fit a model for rate data that avoids the possibility of the dependent variable being negative? It is possible to transform the data to confine the line to positive territory. One way to achieve this is to fit the straight line to the logarithm of the mortality rate rather than to the mortality rate itself.

$$\ln(Y) = a_0 + a_1X_1 + a_2X_2 \tag{10-2}$$

$\ln(Y)$ is the natural logarithm of Y. In equation 10–2, the left side can range from minus infinity to plus infinity, as can the right side, but Y itself must always be positive because one cannot take the logarithm of a negative number. This equation can be solved for Y by taking the antilogarithm of both sides.

$$Y = e^{a_0 + a_1X_1 + a_2X_2} \tag{10-3}$$

Equation 10–3 allows only positive values for Y. On the other hand, to achieve this nicely, we no longer have a simple linear model but an exponential model instead.

Having an exponential model has some implications for the interpretation of the coefficients. Consider again the simple linear model in Figure 10–1. The slope, 0.282 deaths per 100,000 person-years per cigarette per day, is a measure of the absolute amount of increase in the death rate from laryngeal cancer with each additional cigarette smoked per day. If the same type of model were applied to an exposure that was measured on a dichotomous scale, with the value $X = 0$ corresponding to "unexposed" and $X = 1$ corresponding to "exposed," the coefficient

a_1 would represent the rate difference between the exposed and the unexposed.

$$\text{Exposed:} \quad Y_e = a_0 + a_1 X = a_0 + a_1$$

$$\text{Unexposed:} \quad Y_u = a_0 + a_1 X = a_0$$

$$\text{Difference:} \quad Y_e - Y_u = a_1$$

If the equation for the unexposed (when $X = 0$) is subtracted from the equation for the exposed (when $X = 1$), we see that a_1 is the difference in rate between exposed and unexposed. Thus, without any transformation, a_1 can be interpreted as the rate difference between the exposed and unexposed. If, however, we use the logarithmic transformation shown in equations 10–2 and 10–3, we find that the coefficient a_1 in that model is not interpretable as a rate difference.

$$\text{Exposed:} \quad \ln(Y_e) = a_0 + a_1 X = a_0 + a_1$$

$$\text{Unexposed:} \quad \ln(Y_u) = a_0 + a_1 X = a_0$$

$$\text{Difference:} \quad \ln(Y_e) - \ln(Y_u) = a_1$$

$$\text{Ratio:} \quad \frac{Y_e}{Y_u} = e^{a_1}$$

Rather, the antilogarithm of the coefficient (which is what we get when we raise the constant e to the power of the coefficient) is the rate ratio of exposed to unexposed. Thus, the transformation that provides for the good behavior of the predictions from the model with respect to avoiding negative rate estimates also has an implication for the interpretation of the coefficient. Without the transformation, the coefficient estimates rate differences; with the transformation, the coefficient estimates rate ratios (after exponentiating).

Logistic Transformation

Suppose that we had data for which the dependent variable was a risk measure. Whereas rates are never negative but can go as high as infinity, risks are mathematically confined to the small range [0,1]. For any straight line with a nonzero slope, Y ranges from minus infinity to plus infinity rather than from 0 to 1. Consequently, a straight-line model without transformation could lead to individual predicted risk values that are either negative or greater than 1. There is a commonly used transformation, however, the *logistic transformation*, that will confine the predicted risk values to the proper range. It is easier to understand the logistic transformation if we think of it as two transformations. The first converts the risk measure R to a transformed measure that ranges from

0 to infinity instead of [0,1]. This transformation is accomplished by taking $R/(1 - R)$ instead of R. For values of R near 0, the quantity $R/(1 - R)$ will be little different from R; but as R approaches 1, the denominator of the transformed value approaches 0 and the ratio approaches infinity. This transformation stretches the upper end of the range from 1 to infinity. The quantity $R/(1 - R)$ is called the *risk-odds* (any proportion divided by its complement is an odds). The second transformation converts the risk-odds to a measure that ranges all the way from minus infinity to plus infinity. That transformation is the same as the one used above for incidence rates: one simply takes the logarithm of the risk-odds. The resulting measure, after both transformations, is $\ln[R/(1 - R)]$, a quantity that is called a *logit*. The two-step transformation is known as the logistic transformation. The logistic model is one in which the logit is the dependent variable of a straight-line equation.

$$\ln\left[\frac{R}{1 - R}\right] = a_0 + a_1 X \tag{10-4}$$

Equation 10–4 shows a single independent variable, but just as in other linear models, it is possible to add other predictors, making it a multiple logistic model. What is the interpretation of coefficient a_1 in the above model? For an X that is dichotomous, with $X = 1$ for exposed and $X = 0$ for unexposed, the coefficient a_1 is the ratio of logits for exposed to unexposed. This ratio is equal to the logarithm of the risk-odds ratio:

$$\ln\left[\frac{R_1}{1 - R_1}\right] - \ln\left[\frac{R_0}{1 - R_0}\right] = \ln\left[\frac{\dfrac{R_1}{1 - R_1}}{\dfrac{R_0}{1 - R_0}}\right] = \ln\left[\frac{R_1(1 - R_0)}{R_0(1 - R_1)}\right] = a_1 \tag{10-5}$$

This result means that in the logistic model the antilogarithm of the coefficient of a dichotomous exposure term estimates the odds ratio of risks.

$$\frac{R_1(1 - R_0)}{R_0(1 - R_1)} = e^{a_1}$$

As a consequence of the above interpretation for the logistic coefficient, the logistic model has become a popular tool for the analysis of case-control studies, in which the odds ratio is the primary statistic of interest.

Choices among Models

From a mathematical perspective, the advantages of the above transformations are tied to the mathematical behavior of the measures, ensuring that individual estimates from the models conform to the allowed range. From a practical standpoint, however, the transformations dictate what type of measure the coefficients in the model will estimate. If one has risk data and wishes to estimate risk difference, the logistic model will not conveniently provide it; it will provide odds ratios. If one is using a model to obtain risk estimates for people, it may be important to avoid estimates of risk that are negative or greater than 100%, because these are invalid estimates. On the other hand, if the model is being used primarily to assess an overall effect of the exposure from the coefficient in the fitted model, there may be less concern about whether all of the individual estimates stay within their allowable ranges and more interest in which effect measure the model can provide. In many epidemiologic applications, it is the choice among effect measures that dictates the type of model the investigator ought to use.

Consider the data in Table 10–1, which describe the risk of getting

Table 10–1. Risk of developing a hypothetical disease during a 5-year period for 20 subjects

Subject No.	Age (years)	Disease
1	18	0
2	21	0
3	22	0
4	25	0
5	26	0
6	28	0
7	33	0
8	34	0
9	35	0
10	37	0
11	42	1
12	47	1
13	55	0
14	56	1
15	58	0
16	61	1
17	65	1
18	68	1
19	75	1
20	77	1

disease over a 5-year period by the subject's age at the start of the period. Twenty subjects were followed for 5 years, and each either did or did not develop disease. These data are plotted as a scatterplot in Figure 10–2. In a scatterplot with a binary outcome variable that takes values of either 0 or 1, all observations must fall either at 0 or 1 along the vertical axis. Figure 10–2 also shows the linear regression line through the 20 data points and its equation. The intercept of the regression line is the estimated value of the risk for those with age 0. The value of the intercept is -0.49, an impossible value for a risk. In fact, the line estimates a negative risk for all ages below 24 and a risk greater than 100% for all ages greater than 74.

One could avoid the inadmissible risk estimates from the regression line in Figure 10–2 by fitting a logistic model instead of a straight line. The logistic model for the same data is illustrated in Figure 10–3. Its sigmoid shape is characteristic of the logistic curve. This shape keeps the curve within the range [0,1] for any age, preventing the impossible estimates that come from the linear model in Figure 10–2.

It might appear from a comparison of these two figures that the logistic model would always be preferable for risk data, but this example is presented to make the point that the logistic model is not always preferable. The age coefficient in the straight-line equation in Figure 10–2 is interpretable as a risk difference for each year of age: it indicates that the risk increases by an estimated 2% for each year of age. True, the curve would not be expected to fit the data well outside of the central region

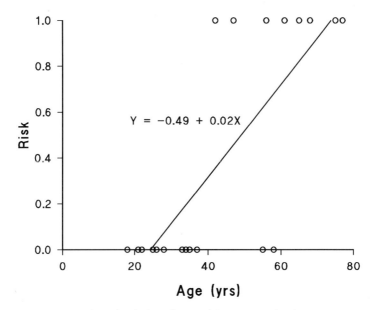

Figure 10–2. Scatterplot of risk data from Table 10–1 and a linear regression line fitted to the data.

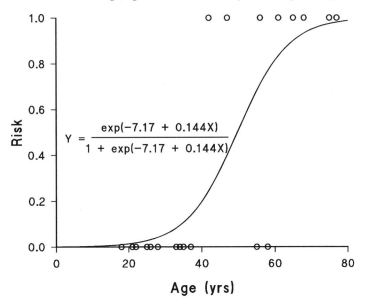

Figure 10–3. Scatterplot of risk data from Table 10–1 and a logistic regression line fitted to the data.

of the graph. Nevertheless, for this region, the straight line provides a simple and useful way of estimating the risk difference for each year of age. In contrast, the logistic model in Figure 10–3 does not permit direct estimation of a risk difference. Instead, it allows estimation of an odds ratio associated with a 1-year increase in age from the antilogarithm of the logistic coefficient: $e^{0.144} = 1.15$, the risk-odds ratio for each 1-year increase in age. Although there is nothing intrinsically wrong with estimating the odds ratio, the straight-line model may be preferable if one wishes to estimate a risk difference. As mentioned above, the logistic model is particularly appropriate for the analysis of case-control data because the odds ratio can be obtained from it and the odds ratio is the statistic of central interest for estimating rate ratios in case-control studies.

The Control of Confounding in Multivariable Analysis

One of the principal advantages of multivariable mathematical models for epidemiologic analysis is the ease with which several confounding variables can be controlled simultaneously. In a multivariable model, the inclusion of several variables results in each term being unconfounded by the other terms. This approach makes it easy and efficient to control confounding by several variables at once, something that might be difficult to achieve through a stratified analysis.

For example, as described in Chapter 8, suppose that were conducting an analysis with five confounding variables, each of which had three categories. To control for these variables in a stratified analysis, we would need to create three strata for the first variable, then divide each of those three strata into three more substrata for the second variable, giving nine strata, and so on until we have $3 \times 3 \times 3 \times 3 \times 3 = 243$ strata. If the variables required more than three categories or if there were more than five variables to control, the number of strata would rise accordingly. With such a large number of strata required for a stratified analysis to control several variables, the data can easily become uninformative because there are too few subjects within strata to give useful estimates. Multivariable analysis solves this problem by allowing a much more efficient way to control for several variables simultaneously. Everything has its price, however, and so it is for multivariable analysis. The price is that the results from a multivariable analysis are more susceptible to bias than those from a stratified analysis.

To illustrate the problem, consider the hypothetical data in Figure 10–4, with data points for exposed and unexposed people by age and by some unspecified but continuous outcome measure. These data show an unfortunate situation in which there is no overlap in the age distribution between the exposed and unexposed populations. If a stratified analysis were undertaken to control for age, there would be little or no overlap in any age category between exposed and unexposed and the stratified analysis would produce no estimate of effect. In essence, a stratified analysis attempting to control for age would give the result that there is no information in the data.

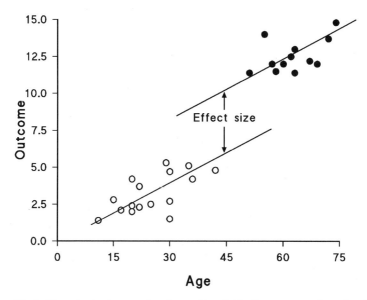

Figure 10–4. Hypothetical example of a multivariable linear regression of a dichotomous exposure and age (*solid circles* are exposed people, and *open circles* are unexposed people).

In contrast, in a multiple regression with both age and exposure terms, the model will essentially fit two parallel lines through the data, one relating age to the outcome for unexposed and the other relating age to the outcome for exposed. If the dichotomous exposure term is coded 0/1, at any age the difference in the outcome between exposed and unexposed is equal to the coefficient for the exposure, which measures the exposure effect.

$$\text{Outcome} = a_0 + a_1 \cdot \text{Exposure} + a_2 \cdot \text{Age}$$

Thus, the multivariable model will produce a statistically stable estimate from the non-overlapping sets of data points. Basically, the model extrapolates the age relation for the unexposed and exposed and estimates the effect from the extrapolated lines, as indicated in Figure 10–4. This estimation process is much more efficient than a stratified analysis, which for these data would not produce any effect estimate at all.

But what if the actual relation between age and the outcome were as pictured in Figure 10–5? If age has the curvilinear relation pictured there, there is no effect of exposure on the outcome and the effect estimated from the model depicted in Figure 10–4 is incorrect. It is simply a bias introduced by the model and its inappropriate extrapolation beyond the observations. Since we cannot know whether the model in Figure 10–4 is appropriate or whether the relation is actually like the pattern depicted in Figure 10–5, the lack of results from the stratified

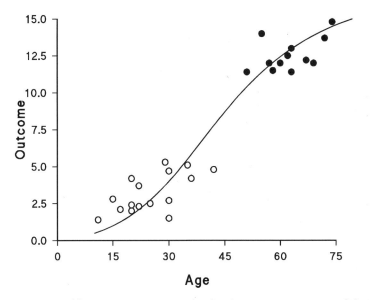

Figure 10–5. Possible age-outcome curve for the data in Figure 10–4 (*solid circles* are exposed people, and *open circles* are unexposed people).

analysis begins to look good compared with the multivariable analysis, which might produce an incorrect result: saying nothing is better than saying something incorrect.

Stratified analysis has other advantages over multivariable analysis. With stratified analysis, both the investigator and the reader (if the stratified data are presented in a paper) are aware of the distribution of the data by the key study variables. In a multivariable analysis, the reader is typically in the dark and the researcher may not be much better off than the reader. For this reason, a multivariable analysis should be used only as a supplement to a stratified analysis, rather than as the primary analytic tool. Unfortunately, many researchers tend to leap into multivariable methods without arming themselves first with the knowledge that would come from a stratified analysis. Typically, the reader is also deprived and presented with no more than the coefficients from the multivariable model. This approach has the lure of seeming sophisticated, but it is a mistake to plunge into multivariable modeling until one has viewed the distribution of the data and analyzed them according to the methods presented in Chapter 8.

Predicting Risk for a Person

Much of the advice on how to construct a multivariable model is crafted for models aimed at making individual predictions of the outcome. For example, Murabito et al.[3] published a logistic model that provided 4-year risk estimates for intermittent claudication (the symptomatic expression of atherosclerosis in the lower extremities). The model is given in table 10–2.

To obtain individual risk estimates from this model, one would multiply the coefficients for each variable in the table by the values for a given person for each variable, which gives the logit for a given person. Because the exponentiated logit equals the risk odds [$\exp(\text{logit}) = R/(1 - R)$], the logit can be converted to a risk estimate by taking into account the relation between risk and risk odds:

$$\text{Odds} = \frac{\text{Risk}}{1 - \text{Risk}} \text{ or Risk} = \frac{\text{Odds}}{1 + \text{Odds}}$$

Thus, the risk can be estimated as $R = \exp(\text{logit})/[1 + \exp(\text{logit})]$. For example, suppose we wish to estimate the risk for a 70-year-old non-smoking man with normal blood pressure, diabetes, coronary heart disease, and a cholesterol level of 250 mg/dl. The logit would be $-8.915 + 1 \cdot 0.503 + 70 \cdot 0.037 + 0 \cdot 0.000 + 1 \cdot 0.950 + 0 \cdot 0.031 + 250 \cdot 0.005 + 1 \cdot 0.994 = -2.628$, and the risk estimate over the next 4 years for intermittent claudication to develop would be $\exp(-2.628)/[1 + \exp(-2.628)] = 6.7\%$. If the man had had stage 2 hypertension instead

Table 10–2. Logistic model to obtain estimates of 4-year risk for intermittent claudication

Variable	Coefficient
Intercept	− 8.915
Male sex	0.503
Age	0.037
Blood pressure	
Normal	0.000
High normal	0.262
Stage 1 hypertension	0.407
Stage 2 + hypertension	0.798
Diabetes	0.950
Cigarettes/day	0.031
Cholesterol (mg/dl)	0.005
Coronary hear disease	0.994

of normal blood pressure, the logit would have been − 1.830 and the risk estimate 13.8%.

In a model such as the one in Table 10–2, the purpose of the individual terms is to improve the estimate of risk. For the purpose of producing a useful risk estimate, it does not matter whether any of the predictor terms is causally related to the outcome. In the model in Table 10–2, some of the predictors cannot be viewed as causes: age is an example of a noncausal predictor, as is heart disease, which presumably does not cause intermittent claudication, although the two diseases may have causes in common. Nevertheless, despite not being causes of intermittent claudication, both age and the presence of coronary heart disease are good predictors of the risk of developing intermittent claudication; therefore, it makes sense to include them in the prediction model. Other predictors, such as cigarette smoking, hypertension, and diabetes, may be causes of intermittent claudication.

Strategy for Constructing Multivariable Models for Epidemiologic Analysis

Although a detailed discussion of the strategy for constructing multivariable models for epidemiologic analysis goes beyond the scope of this book, we outline below some basic principles for the use of these models in causal research.

1. *Do a stratified analysis first.* The first step should always be a stratified analysis. The main contribution of a multivariable analysis to causal research is to enable the simultaneous control of several confounding factors. In accomplishing this goal, multivariable modeling ought to be thought of as a supplement to stratified analysis, to be used

---

Stepwise models in epidemiologic analysis

Stepwise construction of multivariable models uses an algorithm that automatically selects which terms to include in the final model. The algorithm typically selects terms based on the level of statistical significance of the coefficient for each term. Stepwise modeling makes much more sense for the construction of a prediction model than of a causal model. As discussed in Chapter 6, statistical testing does not allow us to grasp either the strength of a relation or the precision of an estimate in isolation; it mixes the two. Using statistical significance levels to choose potential confounders to include in a model is a bad idea, whether it is part of an automatic stepwise algorithm or not, for several reasons. First, the amount of confounding depends on two associations, the relation between the potential confounder and the exposure, and the relation between the potential confounder and the outcome. The coefficient that is tested for significance in a stepwise algorithm evaluates only the relation between the potential confounder and the outcome; it ignores the relation between the potential confounder and the exposure. This method can thus include variables that are not confounding. It can also omit variables that are confounding, but for which the relation with the outcome is not "statistically significant."

---

in situations where there are too many confounders to be handled comfortably in a stratified analysis. Even in those situations, it is common that most of the confounding stems from one or two variables and a multivariable analysis will give essentially the same result as a properly conducted stratified analysis.

2. *Determine which confounders to include in the model.* Start with a set of predictors of the outcome based on the strength of their relation to the outcome, as indicated from analyses of each factor separately or an initial model in which all potential confounders are included. Then, build a model by introducing predictor variables one at a time. After introducing each term, examine the amount of change in the coefficient of the exposure term. If the exposure coefficient changes considerably (most investigators look for a 10% change), then the variable just added to the model is a confounder (provided that it also meets the criteria given on page 108; if not, it is not an important confounder. To judge the confounding effect in this way, it is essential for the exposure to be included in the model as a single term. For example, if the exposure is cigarette smoking, one might enter a single term that quantifies the amount of cigarette smoking rather than several terms for levels of cigarette smoking. It is likewise important to avoid any product terms that involve cigarette smoking (or whatever the exposure variable is) at this stage of the analysis.

3. *Estimate the shape of the exposure–disease relation.* If the exposure is a simple dichotomy, after the confounders are entered into the model, one can estimate the exposure effect directly from the coefficient of the exposure term. If the exposure is a continuous variable, however, such as the number of cigarettes smoked daily, the exposure term will need to be redefined after the confounders are entered into the model. The reason for redefining the exposure term is that the single exposure term that was in the model for the purpose of evaluating confounding will not reveal the shape of the exposure–disease relation for a continuous–exposure variable. If the model involves a logarithmic transformation, as do most of the models commonly used in epidemiologic analysis, a single term for a continuous–exposure variable will be mathematically constrained to take the shape dictated by the model. In a logistic model, the exposure coefficient is the logarithm of the odds ratio for a unit change in the exposure variable. If the exposure is the number of cigarettes smoked daily, the coefficient of a single term that corresponds to the number of cigarettes smoked daily would be the logarithm of the odds ratio for each single cigarette smoked. Because there is only a single term, the model dictates that the effect of each cigarette multiplies the odds ratio by a constant amount. The result is an exponential dose-response curve between exposure and disease (Fig. 10–6).

This exponential shape will be fit to the data regardless of the actual

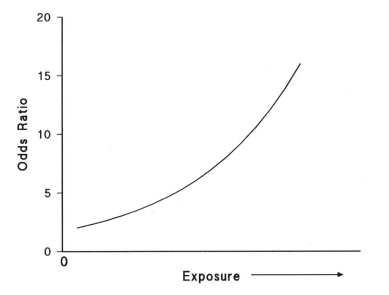

Figure 10–6. Shape of a positive dose-response relation between exposure and disease from a logistic model with a single continuous-exposure term.

shape of the relation between exposure and disease, as long as the exposure variable is continuous and confined to a single term in a model that uses a logarithmic transformation. In linear models, a linear relation, rather than an exponential relation, will be guaranteed. The problem is that the actual relation set by nature may be nothing like the shape of the relation posed by the model. Indeed, few dose-response relations in nature look like the curve in Figure 10–6.

To avoid this difficulty of having the model dictate the shape of the dose-response relation, the investigator can allow the data, rather than the model, to determine the shape of the dose-response relation. To accomplish this goal, the investigator must redefine the exposure term in the model. One popular approach is factoring the exposure: *factoring* refers to categorizing the exposure into ranges and then creating a separate term for each range of exposure, except for one range that becomes the reference value. Thus, cigarette smoking could be categorized into 0, 1–9 cigarettes/day, 10–19 cigarettes/day, and so on. The model would have a term for each cigarette-smoking category except 0, which is the reference category. The variable corresponding to each term would be dichotomous, simply revealing in which category a given person fell. A person would have a value of 1 for the smoking category that applied and a 0 for every other category; a nonsmoker would have a 0 for all smoking categories. The resulting set of coefficients in the fitted model will indicate a separately estimated effect for each level of smoking, determined by the data and not by the mathematics of the model. Another approach for estimating the shape of the dose-response trend is to use curve-smoothing methods, such as *spline regression,* which allow a different fitted curve to apply in different ranges of the exposure variable.

The important point in evaluating dose-response relations is to avoid letting the model determine the shape of the relation between exposure and disease. Whether one uses factoring, splines, or other smoothing methods, it is desirable to allow the data, not the model, to define the shape of the dose-response curve.

4. *Evaluate interaction.* To evaluate interaction appropriately, the investigator should redefine the two exposures in question by considering them jointly as a single composite exposure variable and entering combinations of the exposures into the model as a factored set of terms. For two dichotomous exposures, A and B, the composite variable would have four categories: exposed to neither, exposed to A but not B, exposed to B but not A, and exposed to both. Each person will fall into only one category of the joint exposure to the two variables. Using *exposed to neither* as the reference category, the model will provide estimates of relative effect for each of the other three categories. This method allows use of the multivariable model to estimate departures from additivity, as explained in Chapter 9, without imposing the multiplicative relation implied by the model.[4,5]

Questions

1. In a multivariable model with a nominal scale variable that has three categories, how many indicator terms would need to be included? In general, for a variable with n categories, what is the expression for the number of terms that would need to be included in the model?
2. The analysis depicted in Figure 10–4 is more efficient than a stratified analysis but also more biased. Why is it more biased?
3. Why is an exponential curve, such as the one in Figure 10–6, not a reasonable model for the shape of a dose-response trend? What would be the biologic implication of a dose-response curve that had the shape of the curve in Figure 10–6?
4. If the age term is removed from the model shown in Table 10–2, what would happen to the coefficients for blood pressure? Why?
5. In a multivariable analysis with a continuous-exposure variable, why do we want a single term in the model to evaluate confounding?
6. If we have a continuous-exposure variable and use a single term to evaluate confounding, the shape of the dose-response curve for that term will be implied by the model. We can avoid that imposition by factoring the exposure into several terms defined by categories of exposure. Several exposure terms, however, will make it difficult to evaluate confounding. How can we evaluate confounding and avoid the model-imposed restrictions on the shape of the dose-response curve?

References

1. Kahn, HA: The Dorn study of smoking and mortality among U.S. veterans: report on eight and one-half years of observation. National Cancer Institute Monograph 19. Washington, D.C.: U.S. Department of Health, Education, and Welfare, Public Health Service, 1966.
2. Rothman, KJ, Cann, CI, Flanders, D, et al: Epidemiology of laryngeal cancer. *Epidemiol Rev* 1980;2:195–209.
3. Murabito, JM, D'Agostino, RB, Sibershatz, H, et al: Intermittent claudication. A risk profile from the Framingham Heart Study. *Circulation* 1997; 96:44–49.
4. Rothman, KJ: *Modern Epidemiology*, 1st ed. Boston: Little, Brown, 1986.
5. Assman, SF, Hosmer, DW, Lemeshow, S, et al: Confidence intervals for measures of interaction. *Epidemiology* 1996;7:286–290.

11

Epidemiology in Clinical Settings

Clinical epidemiology focuses the application of epidemiologic principles on questions that relate to diagnosis, prognosis, and therapy. It also encompasses screening and other aspects of preventive medicine at both the population and the individual levels. Therapeutic thinking has been greatly affected by advances in pharmacoepidemiology, an area that has extended the reach of epidemiologic research from the study of drug benefits to that of adverse effects and has led to the burgeoning field of *outcomes research*. Outcomes research marries epidemiologic methods with clinical decision theory to determine which therapeutic approaches are the most cost-effective. In all of these areas of medicine and preventive medicine, the role of epidemiology is becoming more and more prominent.

Diagnosis

Assigning a diagnosis is both crucial and subtle. To a large extent, diagnosis may appear to involve intuition, conviction, and guesswork, processes that are opaque to quantification and analysis. Nevertheless, formal approaches to understanding and refining the steps in assigning a diagnosis have helped to clarify the thinking and solidify the foundation for diagnostic decision-making. The basis for formulating a diagnosis comprises the data from signs, symptoms, and diagnostic test results that distinguish those with a specific disease from those who do not have that disease.

The Gold Standard

Diagnosis cannot be a perfect process. Rarely does any sign or symptom, or any combination of them, distinguish completely between those with and those without a disease. Often, a diagnosis is considered established when a specific combination of signs and symptoms that has been posed as the criterion for disease is present. A diagnosis meeting this standard may be "definitive" but only in a circular sense, that is, by definition. Another way that a definitive diagnosis can be reached is by expert judgment, often by consensus; but once again, this approach makes a diagnosis definitive only by definition. No approach is perfect, and two different approaches to the same disease will not necessarily lead to the same classification for every patient. Nevertheless, even if it is arbitrary, we need to have some definition of disease to use as a 'gold standard' by which we can judge the performance of individual signs and symptoms or screening tests.

Sensitivity and Specificity

For years the diagnosis of tuberculosis has rested on detection of the *Mycobacterium tuberculosis* organism from smears of acid-fast bacilli and from culture, but this method requires 10,000 bacteria/ml and does not distinguish among various mycobacteria.[1] Catanzaro et al.[1] reported how well an acid-fast smear predicted the diagnosis of clinical tuberculosis among patients suspected of having active pulmonary tuberculosis on the sole basis of clinical judgment. The diagnosis of tuberculosis was established by an expert panel of three judges, who used culture information and clinical information according to specific guidelines to classify patients into those who had and those who did not have tuberculosis. Among the 338 patients enrolled, the distribution by diagnosis and by outcome of the acid-fast smear results is given in Table 11-1.

From the data in Table 11-1, we see that 72/338 (21%) patients suspected of having active pulmonary tuberculosis were diagnosed as having it. Among the 72 tuberculosis patients, 43 (60%) had a positive smear. This proportion is known as the *sensitivity* of the smear. The sensitivity of a test, sign, or symptom is defined as the proportion of people with the disease who also have a positive result for the test, sign, or symptom. If everyone who has the disease has a given sign or symptom, the sensitivity of that sign or symptom would be 100%. It is easy to find signs or symptoms that have high sensitivities. For example, in diagnosing headache, we might note that all patients have heads, making its sensitivity 100%. Having a head would have a low *specificity*, however. The specificity of a test, sign, or symptom is the proportion of people among those who do not have the disease who have a negative test, sign, or symptom. The specificity of the acid-fast smear test, based on the data in Table 11-1, was 244/266 (92%). The specificity of having a head in diagnosing a headache would be 0, because everyone has a head. The most useful tests, signs, or symptoms for diagnosing a disease are those with both high sensitivity and high specificity. A test with 100% sensitivity and 100% specificity would be positive for everyone with disease and negative for everyone without disease. Most tests do not provide such a distinct separation of those with and without disease.

Tests, signs, and symptoms can be used in combination to improve either sensitivity or specificity. Suppose test A had a sensitivity of 80% and a specificity of 90% by itself, and test B also had a sensitivity of 80% and a specificity of 90%. If we used the two tests in combination to

Table 11-1. Distribution of patients suspected of having active pulmonary tuberculosis by diagnosis and results of acid-fast bacillus smear*

Smear	Tuberculosis	No Tuberculosis	Total
Positive	43	22	65
Negative	29	244	273
Total	72	266	338

Sensitivity of smear $= \dfrac{43}{72} = 60\%$ Predictive value positive of smear $= \dfrac{43}{65} = 66\%$

Specificity of smear $= \dfrac{244}{266} = 92\%$ Predictive value negative of smear $= \dfrac{244}{273} = 89\%$

*Data from Catanzaro et al.[1]

indicate disease, we might postulate that it would require a positive result on both tests to indicate the presence of disease. If the test results were independent of each other, then $0.8 \times 0.8 = 0.64$ of all patients with disease would test positive on both, making the sensitivity of the combination 64%, worse than the sensitivity of either test alone. On the other hand the specificity would improve because those who are negative for the combination would include all of those who tested negative on either test: 90% of those without disease would test negative on the first test, and of the 10% who did not, 90% would test negative on the second test, making the specificity of the combination $0.9 + (0.1 \times 0.9) = 99\%$. Thus, requiring a positive result from two tests increases the specificity but decreases the sensitivity.

The reverse occurs if a positive result on either test is taken to indicate the presence of disease: for the example given, 80% of those with disease would test positive for the first test and of the remaining 20%, 80% would test positive on the second test, making the sensitivity $0.8 + (0.2 \times 0.8) = 96\%$. The price paid to obtain a higher sensitivity is a lower specificity, which would be the proportion of those without disease who test negative on both tests, $0.9 \times 0.9 = 81\%$.

This discussion assumes that the test results are independent, which will rarely be the case. Nevertheless, the principle will always apply that combinations of tests, signs, and symptoms can be used to increase either sensitivity or specificity at the cost of the other, depending on how a positive outcome for the combination of tests is defined. This principle is used to detect cervical cancer by a Pap smear, which has a high sensitivity but a low specificity. As a result, a Pap smear will detect nearly all cervical cancers but has a high proportion of false-positives. By requiring a sequence of positive Pap smears before taking further diagnostic action, however, it is possible to improve the specificity of the smear (that is, reduce the false-positives) without compromising the already high sensitivity much. Recent work has led to an improvement on the approach of repeated smears: now, a single cervical smear can be simultaneously tested for the DNA of human papillomavirus, another risk factor for cervical cancer, to improve the specificity of a single screen rather than having to rely on repeat Pap testing.[2]

Predictive Value

Sensitivity and specificity describe the characteristics of a test, sign, or symptom in correctly classifying those who have or do not have a disease. *Predictive value* is a measure of the usefulness of a test, sign, or symptom in classifying people with disease. It can be calculated from the same basic data used to calculate sensitivity and specificity. Consider the tuberculosis example in Table 11–1. We can use these data to calculate the predictive value of a positive smear. Among the 65 people with a positive smear, 43 had tuberculosis. Thus, a positive smear correctly indicated the presence of tuberculosis in 43/65 (66%) people who were tested. This proportion is referred to as the *predictive value positive*, or the predictive value of a positive test, usually abbreviated as PV^+. We can also measure the predictive value negative, or the predictive value of a negative test, which is abbreviated PV^-. In the same data, of the 273 who had a negative smear, 244 did not have tuberculosis, making the PV^- of the smear 244/273 (89%).

Sensitivity and specificity should theoretically be constant properties of a test, regardless of the population being tested, although in practice, they can vary with the mix of patients. Predictive value, in contrast, varies even theoretically from one population to another because it is highly dependent on the prevalence of disease in the population being tested. We can illustrate the dependence of predictive value on the prevalence of disease by examining what would result if we added to the population described in Table 11–1 500 people who did not have tuberculosis. The effect is similar to the change one would find in moving from a clinic serving a population in which tuberculosis was common to a clinic serving a population in which tuberculosis was less common. The augmented data are displayed in Table 11–2.

Let us assume that the sensitivity and specificity of the test remain the same. We still have 72 people with tuberculosis, of whom 43 will show a positive smear. We now have 766 people without tuberculosis, of whom 703 will have a negative smear, giving the same specificity as before, 92%. The PV^+ and PV^- are considerably different in this second population, however. The PV^+ is 43/106 = 41%, much less than the 66% from Table 11–1. As the prevalence of disease decreases, the PV^+ will decrease as well. At the same time, the PV^- has changed from 89% in the original data to 703/732 = 96% in the augmented data. As the prevalence of the disease decreases, the PV^+ decreases but the PV^- increases.

These changes in predictive value with changes in prevalence should

Table 11–2. Data from Table 11–1 augmented by 500 people without tuberculosis

Smear	Tuberculosis	No Tuberculosis	Total
Positive	43	63	106
Negative	29	703	732
Total	72	766	838

$$\text{Sensitivity of smear} = \frac{43}{72} = 60\% \quad \text{Predictive value positive of smear} = \frac{43}{106} = 41\%$$

$$\text{Specificity of smear} = \frac{703}{766} = 92\% \quad \text{Predictive value negative of smear} = \frac{703}{732} = 96\%$$

not be too surprising. If we tested a population in which no one had disease, there would still be some false-positive test results. The PV^+ of these results would be 0 because no one in that population actually had the disease. On the other hand the PV^- would be perfect if no one in the population had the disease. Taking the other extreme, if everyone in a population had the disease, then the PV^+ would be 100% and the PV^- would be 0. Changes in predictive value with the prevalence of disease have implications for the use of diagnostic and screening tests. Tests that may have reasonably good PV^+ in a clinic population presenting with symptoms may have little PV^+ in an asymptomatic population being screened for disease. Therefore, it may not make sense to convert diagnostic tests into screening tests that would be applied to populations with few signs or symptoms of disease and, consequently, a low prevalence of disease.

Screening

The premise of screening is that for many diseases early detection improves the prognosis. Otherwise, there is no point to screening, because it is expensive both in monetary terms and in terms of the burden it places on the screened population. To be suitable for screening, a disease must be detectable during a preclinical phase by some test, and early treatment should convey a benefit over treatment at the time when the disease would have come to attention without screening.[3] Furthermore, the benefit that early treatment conveys should exceed the cost of screening. These costs are more than just the expense of administering the screening test to a healthy population. Screening will result in some false-positive results, saddling those who have the false result with the mistaken prospect of facing a disease that they do not have. Furthermore, a false-positive result will usually lead to further tests and sometimes even treatments that are unnecessary and risky. Another cost comes from false-negative results, which provide false reassurance about the absence of disease. Even for those whom the screening test labels correctly with disease, there is a psychological cost that comes from being labeled earlier in the natural history of the process than would have occurred without screening. Balancing this cost is the useful reassurance for those who do not have the disease that comes from having tested negative.

For screening to succeed, the disease being screened should have a reasonably long preclinical phase so that the prevalence of people in this preclinical phase is high. If the pre-clinical phase is short and people who develop the disease promptly pass through it into a clinical phase, there is little point to screening. In such a situation, the low prevalence of the preclinical phase in the population will produce a low PV^+ for the screening test.

Because screening advances the date of diagnosis for a disease, it can be difficult to measure its effect. Suppose the disease is cancer. The success of treating cancer is usually measured in terms of the survival time after diagnosis or the time to recurrence. If early treatment is advantageous, one would expect it to result in longer survival times or longer times until recurrence. After screening, however, survival times and times to recurrence will increase even if the screening and earlier treatment do no good. The reason is that the time of diagnosis is moved ahead by screening, so the diagnosis is registered earlier in the natural history of the disease process than it would have been without screening. The difference in time between the date of diagnosis with screening and the date of diagnosis without screening is called the *lead time*. Lead time should not be counted as part of the survival time after disease diagnosis, since it does not represent any real benefit. If it is counted, it erroneously inflates the survival time, a problem known as *lead-time bias.*

In addition to lead-time bias, another difficulty in evaluating the success of a screening effort is bias that comes from self-selection of subjects who decide to be screened. This bias is called *prognostic selection bias.* Because screening programs are voluntary, those who volunteer to get screened will differ in many ways from those who refuse to be screened. Volunteers are likely to be more interested in their health, to be more eager to take actions that improve their health, and to have a more favorable clinical course even in the absence of a benefit from screening. One way to avoid this bias, as well as lead-time bias and the effect of length-biased sampling (see box), is to evaluate the screening test or program by conducting a randomized trial. In nonexperimental studies, however, these biases are important issues that must be taken into account to obtain a valid assessment of screening efficacy.

Prognosis

Prognosis is a qualitative or quantitative prediction of the outcome of an illness. A full description of the prognosis involves not merely the dura-

Length-biased sampling

Another difficulty in measuring the effect of screening comes from *length-biased sampling,* which results from natural variability in the progression rate of disease. To simplify the issue, suppose that breast cancer comes in two types, fast-progressing and slow-progressing. Those with fast-progressing breast cancer have the worse prognosis; their disease goes quickly through the preclinical phase into a clinical phase and spreads rapidly, leading to an early demise for many patients. Slow-progressing breast cancer, however, is more benign, taking many more months or years to progress through the preclinical phase into a clinical phase that also is characterized by slow progression. Women with slow-progressing breast cancer will have a better prognosis, even without treatment, although they are also more likely to benefit from treatment.

Let us assume that an equal number of cases of slow-progressing and fast-progressing breast cancer occurred in a population. Despite the equal incidence, the prevalence of slow-progressing cases would be greater because prevalence reflects duration as well as incidence. Thus, there will be more slow-progressing cases in the preclinical phase of disease, because each case takes longer to pass through that stage of the disease process. A screening program, therefore, would tend to identify more slow-progressing cases than fast-progressing cases. Even if early identification and treatment of breast cancer had no effect on the disease, cases identified in a screening program would tend to have a better prognosis than the average of all cases because of length-biased sampling, since the screening tends to favor identifying slow-progressing cases with a better prognosis.

tion of the illness and the timing of recovery or progression but also the nature of the illness as it progresses along its clinical course. Epidemiologic evaluation of prognosis, however, focuses on the measurement in epidemiologic terms of serious sequelae or recovery. The most serious sequela is death, and much of epidemiologic prognostication focuses on the occurrence of death among newly diagnosed or treated patients.

The simplest epidemiologic measure of prognosis is the *case fatality rate.* Despite the name, this measure is an incidence proportion rather than a true rate. It is the proportion of newly diagnosed cases that die from the disease. Strictly speaking, the case fatality rate should be measured over a fixed and stated time period. For example, we could give the case fatality rate measured over a 3-month or 12-month period. Traditionally, however, the measure has been used to describe the clinical course of acute infectious illnesses that would progress toward recovery or death within a short time. The time period implicit in the measure refers to the period of the active infection and its aftermath and is often left unspecified. Thus, we might describe typhoid fever as having a case fatality rate of 0.01, paralytic poliomyelitis as having a case fatality rate of 0.05, and Ebola disease as having a case fatality rate of 0.75, each with its own characteristic time period during which the patient either dies or recovers.[4] Eventually, of course, all patients with any disease will die from one cause or another. The presumption of the case fatality rate is that essentially all of the deaths that occur promptly after disease onset are a consequence of the disease.

For diseases that run a clinical course over long periods, it becomes more important to specify the time period over which case fatality is measured. When case fatality is measured over longer time periods, the term *case fatality rate* is often not even used. Instead, we use terms such as *5-year survival* to refer to the proportion surviving for 5 years after diagnosis, which is simply the complement of the proportion who die during the 5 years. Beyond a simple incidence proportion or survival proportion, we can derive a survival curve, which gives the survival probability according to time since diagnosis. The survival curve conveys information about the survival proportion for all time periods up to the limit of what has been observed, thus providing greater information than any single survival proportion. (A common method for obtaining a survival curve is the *Kaplan-Meier product-limit method,* which is a variant of the life-table approach described in Chapter 3. The Kaplan-Meier approach recalculates the proportion that survives at the time of each death in a cohort.[5])

The complement and close cousin to the survival curve is the curve that expresses the cumulative proportion who succumb to a specific end point. Figure 11–1 exemplifies a pair of such cumulative incidence curves, which describe the results of a randomized trial that compared the effect of ramipril, an angiotensin-converting enzyme inhibitor, and placebo at preventing the occurrence of myocardial infarction, stroke, or death in patients with certain cardiovascular risk factors.[6] In this example, the curves show the cumulative proportion who experienced any of the end points over a 5-year follow-up period.

Therapy

It has been said that it was not until the early twentieth century that the average patient visiting the average physician stood to benefit from the encounter. The course of illness today is often greatly affected by the choice of treatment options. The large clinical research enterprise that evaluates new therapies is heavily dependent on epidemiology. In fact, a large part of clinical research is clinical epidemiology.

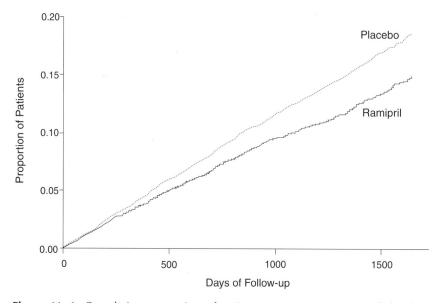

Figure 11–1. Cumulative proportion of patients experiencing myocardial infarction, stroke, or death from cardiovascular causes, by treatment group[6] (adapted with permission from the *New England Journal of Medicine,* copyright © 2000, Massachusetts Medical Society. All rights reserved).

Clinical Trials

The randomized clinical trial is the epidemiologic centerpiece of clinical epidemiology. Though the clinical trial is but one type of epidemiologic experiment (the others are field trials and community intervention trials), it is by far the most common. (See Chapter 4 for a discussion of the types of epidemiologic experiment.) A full discussion of clinical trials merits a separate textbook; here, we only touch on some highlights that bear on the interpretation of trial results.

The central advantage of trials over nonexperimental studies is their ability to control confounding effectively. A particularly knotty problem in therapeutics is *confounding by indication.* When nonexperimental studies are conducted to compare the outcomes of different treatments, confounding by indication can present an insuperable problem. Confounding by indication is a bias that stems from inherent differences in prognosis between patients given different therapies. For example, suppose a new antibiotic shows promise in treating resistant strains of meningitis-causing bacteria, but has common adverse effects and is costly. It is likely that the new treatment will be reserved for patients who face the greatest risk of a fatal outcome. Even if the drug is highly effective, the mortality rate among those who receive it could be greater than that among those receiving the standard drugs because those who get the new drug are at the highest risk. A valid evaluation of the new drug can be achieved only if the prognostic differences can be adjusted or otherwise controlled in the epidemiologic comparison. Although nonexperimental studies can deal with such confounding by indication if there is sufficiently good information on risk factors for the disease complication that the therapy aims to prevent, the best efforts to control it will often fail to remove all of the bias. This problem is the primary motivation to conduct experiments that compare therapies. With the random assignment that is possible in a clinical trial, prognostic factors can be balanced between groups receiving different therapies.

Assessing baseline imbalances in clinical trials
Baseline risk factors are prognostic factors for the outcome that are measured at the time of random assignment. If randomization succeeds in achieving its goal, the frequency of the outcome would be similar in the treatment groups created by randomization, apart from the effect of the intervention. Although there is no direct way to measure whether such a balance in overall prognosis for the treatment groups has been achieved, it is possible to measure the distribution of individual prognostic factors in the compared groups to see how well balanced these are. Any imbalance in a baseline risk factor represents confounding, because a confounding factor is a risk factor associated with exposure. To say that a risk factor is imbalanced means that it is not distributed equally in the compared treatment groups, and therefore it is associated with the assigned treatment.

Randomization is intended to prevent confounding. The outcome of a random process, however, is predictable only if aggregated over many repetitions. In a specific case or a particular trial, unlikely distributions can result from the randomization. In the University Group Diabetes Program,[7] the group randomly assigned to receive tolbutamide was older on average than the group randomly assigned to receive placebo. Thus, there was confounding by age in the evaluation of the tolbutamide effect. This age confounding is illustrated in Tables 5-3 and 5-4: the crude difference in mortality proportion between tolbutamide and placebo, ignoring the age imbalance, was 0.045 in Table 5-3, whereas after stratifying into two age groups in Table 5-4, the tolbutamide effect was estimated to be 0.035.

Two distributions will rarely be identical, so how can we tell when the imbalance in a baseline risk factor is severe enough to warrant treating the variable as a confounding factor? If a factor that is severely imbalanced has only a small effect on the outcome, there will be little confounding even with the severe imbalance. On the other hand, even a minor imbalance in a strong risk factor for the outcome might lead to worrisome confounding. Thus, the amount of imbalance in the risk factor by itself is not a good guide to the amount of confounding that the imbalance introduces. The way to assess the confounding is to use the same approach that epidemiologists use in other situations, which is basically the method used to compare the effects of tolbutamide estimated in Tables 5–3 and 5–4. By comparing the crude estimate of effect, obtained without control of confounding, with an unconfounded estimate, one can see how much confounding is removed when the variable is treated as a confounder. That is the best way to measure the amount of confounding caused by the baseline imbalance. It may seem cumbersome that one has to control the confounding to measure how much there is, but no evaluation of the imbalance in the baseline risk factor alone can reveal the amount of confounding, which depends on the interplay between that imbalance and the relation of the risk factor to the outcome.

A nearly universal mistake in conducting and reporting clinical trials is to use statistical significance testing to assess imbalances in baseline risk factors. Chapter 6 explains the problems with statistical significance testing in general and suggests that it be avoided. Table 6–3 gives the results from a prominent clinical trial that was misinterpreted because the authors relied on statistical significance for their inference. Using statistical significance to interpret the results of a study is undesirable, but it is even less desirable to use statistical significance to assess baseline differences in a trial. Aside from the usual problems with statistical significance testing described in Chapter 6, using testing to assess baseline imbalances introduces further problems. Perhaps the most obvious is that an imbalance in baseline risk factors by itself does not reflect the amount of confounding, as explained above. A second problem is that the amount of confounding is the result of the strength of the associations between the baseline risk factor and the two main study variables, treatment (exposure) and outcome (disease). In contrast, the result of a statistical significance test depends not just on the strength of the association being tested but also on the size of the study: for a given strength of association, the more data, the smaller the p value. Thus, a given amount of confounding in a large study might yield statistically significant differences in a baseline risk factor, but the same amount of confounding in a small study might not yield a statistically significant difference in the baseline risk factor. For these reasons, it does not make much sense to use statistical significance testing to evaluate confounding. Instead, one should simply compare the crude effect estimate with the estimate after controlling for the possible confounder and assess the difference between the two results.

Dealing with baseline imbalances in clinical trials
If an imbalance of baseline risk factors is serious enough to induce worrisome confounding into the effect estimate of a trial, how should it be handled? One school of thought holds that any imbalance should be ignored because the intent of a randomized trial is to compare the experience of the randomized groups, period. According to this theory, one

---

An unrejectable null hypothesis

There is yet another reason that the use of statistical significance testing to evaluate baseline imbalances in a clinical trial makes no sense. If such a statistical test is applied (and it is unfortunately applied in nearly every published trial), one might ask what null hypothesis it tests. The answer must be that the null hypothesis is that any observed imbalance is just the result of chance. If a statistically significant result is observed, one would ordinarily take that to mean that the null hypothesis is rejected. In the case of baseline imbalances in a randomized trial, that would mean rejecting the hypothesis that chance produced the imbalances. But we cannot reject that hypothesis! Apart from chicanery or incompetence, we know that chance did in fact produce the imbalance: the imbalance is the result of a randomized allocation. Random assignment can produce unusual results, but we already know in a trial that the imbalances that do occur are due to chance. Therefore, it makes no sense to test the null hypothesis. Actually, it makes no difference whether the imbalance was caused by chance or not. What matters is that the imbalance exists, and what is important to know is how much confounding it causes. Statistical significance testing cannot reveal that, but the straightforward application of epidemiologic rules for assessing confounding can.

---

simply hopes that randomization will control successfully for all possible confounding factors, and then one relies on conducting a crude analysis without any control of confounding, no matter what happens after the randomization. The motivation for this view is that if the researcher does control for confounding, problems can be introduced into the analysis that can nullify the benefits of random assignment.

It is true that in an ideal setting randomization will prevent confounding. But if randomization has failed to prevent confounding, the options that the investigator faces are either to rely on a biased comparison of the crude data or to conduct an analysis that controls for the confounding that has been identified. Given the expense and effort of a trial, it makes little sense to ignore confounding that has been identified and risk having the results of the study ignored because critics claim that the study is biased. It makes much more sense to attempt to control for any confounding that has been identified. Critics may still claim that the randomization has "failed" (although it has not really failed). Nevertheless, the hope that random assignment will prevent confounding has already been defeated if confounding has been identified in the data. The question is how to proceed now that randomization has not prevented confounding. Some might argue that if an identified confounder is controlled, that process itself can introduce confounding by some other, possibly unidentified factor. Although that is possible, there is no basis to assume that control of a known bias will introduce an unknown bias. Instead, it is more reasonable to control all identified confounders and treat the analysis like any other epidemiologic study.[8,9]

Example: the Alzheimer's disease cooperative study of selegiline and α-tocopherol

The question of how to deal with baseline differences arose in a trial of selegiline and α-tocopherol, two treatments intended to slow progression of Alzheimer's disease.[10] The trial used a factorial design of two treatments. In a factorial design, participants are assigned to groups so that every combination of treatments is studied. With two treatments, there will be four groups. In this study, one group received only α-tocopherol, one group received only selegiline, one group received both α-tocopherol and selegiline, and one group received a placebo. The mean score on the Mini-Mental State Examination of the patients randomly assigned to receive α-tocopherol alone was 11.3 on a scale from 0 to 30, whereas the placebo group had a mean score of 13.3; higher scores are better. Thus, the random assignment resulted in the group assigned to α-tocopherol having lower cognitive function at baseline than the placebo group. At first, the investigators disregarded this difference and found that the α-tocopherol group had a risk ratio of 0.7 with respect to the occurrence of at least one of several primary end points, including death, institutionalization, and onset of severe dementia. Thus, the estimate of the crude effect of α-tocopherol showed a substantial benefit. We would expect that adjusting for the baseline difference in the Mini-Mental State Examination would have increased the estimated benefit even further because the α-tocopherol group had more signs of dementia to begin with. That was the case; after adjustment for baseline differences, the estimated risk ratio was 0.47, showing an even greater benefit.

These findings were challenged by a correspondent,[11] who claimed that the adjusted results were biased. The critic did not offer a clear rationale for the supposed bias, nor did he discuss its magnitude or direction. When a critic suggests that a result is biased, it is incumbent on him or her to quantify the effect of the bias. In this case, the critic implied that the adjusted results should be ignored and that the results from the crude analysis should be used for interpretation. Recall that even the crude effect, with no adjustment for the baseline difference, showed a worthwhile benefit, with a risk ratio of 0.70, indicating a 30% reduction in the occurrence of the primary end-point events. Nevertheless, the critic said that "no true effect of treatment has been proved," suggesting that α-tocopherol had no effect at all. This conclusion was apparently based not on the effect estimate, which showed a 30% reduction in occurrence of the adverse end points, but rather on a lack of statistical significance. This misinterpretation of the findings was aided by authors of the original report, who themselves placed great emphasis on statistical significance. They also assessed the baseline differences in terms of their statistical significance, rather than in terms of the amount of confounding that they produced.

In this example, which estimate of effect should we rely on as the best estimate of the effect of α-tocopherol on Alzheimer's disease? The crude estimate for the risk ratio is 0.70, and the adjusted estimate is 0.47; but we know that the crude estimate is biased because of baseline differences on the Mini-Mental State Examination. It does not matter what the p value is for these baseline differences, nor exactly how they arose; what matters is the amount of confounding that they introduce. Contrary to what the correspondent asserted, the estimate of the α-tocopherol effect, after adjusting for those baseline differences, has less bias, not more bias, than the crude estimate of the effect. With adjustment, the estimated benefit of α-tocopherol in slowing the progression of Alzheimer's disease is striking. Unfortunately, in this example, distrust for analyses that remove confounding and reliance on statistical significance testing for interpretation called into question a striking benefit.

Blinding and use of placebos in clinical trials

Blinding refers to hiding information about treatment assignment from the key participants in a trial. The concern is that knowledge of the treatment will influence the evaluation of the outcome. This concern relates most directly to the person or persons who are supposed to make judgments or decisions regarding the outcome. If the outcome is hospitalization for an exacerbation of the disease, for example, the physician who makes the determination about hospitalization might be influenced by knowledge about which treatment was assigned to a given patient. This concern is amplified if the physician has a strong view about the merits of the new therapy. If the physician does not know which treatment the patient has received, then the evaluation should be free of this source of potential bias.

Blinding is not always necessary. If the only outcome of interest is death, as opposed to hospitalization, there is little reason to be concerned about biased classification of the outcome, because judgment is not an important factor in determining whether someone is dead. Blinding may not always be feasible, either. If the treatment is an elaborate intervention, such as major surgery, it may not be feasible or ethical to provide a sham procedure that would make blinding possible. Thus, although blinding is often desirable, it is not always necessary or possible.

Some trials are described as *double-blind*. This term implies that the evaluator assessing the patient for the possible outcome does not know the treatment assignment and that the patient also does not know the treatment assignment. It may be that the person who administers the

Ethics of placebo use in randomized trials

Only decades ago, it was common for physicians to prescribe placebos so that patients could benefit from improved expectations. Today, such practice is rare, and many would consider it unethical. Placebo use continues today in randomized trials, however, where the biggest concern remains ethical. According to the Declaration of Helsinki,[13] the interests of patients must come before the interests of science and society. Furthermore, every patient in a trial should be assured of getting the equivalent of the best available treatment, even those assigned to the comparison group. Therefore, it is unethical to use a placebo in any trial if there is already an accepted treatment for the condition under study. Instead, an investigator must test a new therapy against the existing standard, to see if it beats the current best treatment. According to the principles embodied in the Declaration of Helsinki, no researcher should deny a patient the best available treatment solely for the purpose of learning whether a new treatment is better than placebo. Identifying new treatments that are better than placebo but worse than the current best treatment is of less interest than identifying new treatments that are better than existing treatments. As medicine progresses, there should be fewer and fewer conditions for which a placebo-controlled study is ethical because there will be standard therapies that are better than placebo for more and more conditions. Unfortunately, the use of placebos in trials has achieved paradigm status in the minds of many researchers and even official agencies.[14] The paradigm should certainly include a comparison, but not necessarily a placebo comparison.

treatment is also kept unaware of which treatment is being assigned, in which case the study might be described as *triple-blind*. In all of these situations, the goal is to keep the information about treatment assignment a secret so that evaluation of the outcome will not be affected.

One method often used to facilitate blinding is a placebo treatment for the comparison group. A placebo treatment is intended to have no biologic effect outside of the offer of treatment itself. Placebo pills typically contain sugar or other essentially inert ingredients. Such pills can be manufactured to be indistinguishable from the new therapy being offered. Other types of placebo treatment could involve sham procedures. For example, a trial of acupuncture could involve as a placebo treatment the use of acupuncture needles at points that are, according to acupuncture theory, not correct. Placebo treatments need to be adapted to the individual experiment in which they are used.

Although the use of a placebo facilitates blinding, this is not the primary reason to use a placebo. It has long been known that even if a treatment has no effect, offering that treatment may have a salubrious effect. An offer of treatment is an offer of hope, and it may bring the expectation of treatment success. Expectations are thought to have a powerful influence on outcome. If so, a new treatment may have an effect that comes only through the lifting of patient expectations. According to some scientists, "the history of medical treatment until recently is largely the history of the placebo effect." [12] The use of a placebo comparison in a trial is intended to distinguish new treatments that have no more than the placebo effect from those that have more of an effect. The placebo effect itself is highly variable, depending on the nature of the outcome and the nature of the treatment.

Pharmacoepidemiology

Drug epidemiology, also known as *pharmacoepidemiology,* is an active area of epidemiologic research that focuses mostly on the safety of therapeutic drugs. Because adverse effects are typically much less common than the intended effects of drugs, randomized trials conducted to evaluate the efficacy of new drugs are seldom large enough to provide an adequate assessment of drug safety. Consequently, most of the epidemiologic information on drug safety comes from studies conducted after a drug is marketed.

This research activity is usually referred to as *postmarketing surveillance.* Much of it is not surveillance in the traditional sense but, instead, based on discrete studies aimed at evaluating specific hypotheses. In the United States, however, the Food and Drug Administration (FDA) encourages the voluntary reporting of suspected adverse drug effects. These "spontaneous reports" are challenging to interpret. First, only a small, but unknown, proportion of suspected adverse drug effects are reported spontaneously; presumably, unexpected deaths, liver or kidney failure, and other serious events are more likely to be reported than skin rashes, but even so it is widely believed that only a small fraction of serious events are reported spontaneously. Second, it is difficult to know whether the number of reported exposed cases, who represent only one cell in a 2 × 2 table of exposure versus disease, represent an actual excess of exposed cases or just the number that chance would predict. Despite these problems, adept analysis of spontaneous reports has proved to be a useful surveillance method, often triggering more formal evaluations of possible adverse effects.

Case reports such as those reported to the FDA as part of their surveillance effort are presumed to represent cases that are attributed to a given drug exposure; that is, the reporting process requires the reporter to make an inference about whether a specific drug exposure caused the adverse event. This type of inference, while encouraged in clinical practice, runs counter to the thinking that prevails in an epidemiologic study. As discussed in Chapter 2, it is not possible to infer logically whether a specific factor was the cause of an observed event. We can only theorize about the causal connection and test our theories with data. In epidemiology, we typically collect data from many people before making inferences about a causal connection, and we usually do not apply the inference to any specific person. If a person receives a drug and promptly dies of anaphylactic shock, a causal inference about the connection between the drug and the death may appear strong; but many inferences for individual observations are tenuous, based more on conviction than anything else. The danger of thinking in terms of causal inferences on individuals is that if this approach is applied to epidemiologic data, it defeats the validity of the epidemiologic process. If case inclusion in any epidemiologic evaluation takes into account information on exposure, it is apt to lead to biases. Instead, disease should be defined on the basis of criteria that have nothing to do with exposure, and the inferences in an epidemiologic study should relate to the general causal theory rather than what happened in any single person.

One way in which this problem can get out of hand is if a disease is defined in terms of an exposure. Once that occurs, a valid epidemiologic evaluation may be impossible. Consider the example of "analgesic nephropathy." This "disease" refers to kidney failure that is supposedly induced by the effect of analgesic drugs, based on the theory that analgesic drugs cause kidney failure in some people. Although there may be no reason to doubt the theory, if it is applied by defining cases of analgesic nephropathy to be kidney failure in people who have taken analgesics for a specified time, it will be impossible to evaluate epidemiologically the relation of analgesics to kidney failure. A valid evaluation would require that kidney failure be defined and diagnosed on the basis of disease-related criteria alone and that information about analgesic use be excluded from the disease definition and diagnosis. Even if the disease is not called analgesic nephropathy, as long as the information on analgesic use is taken into account in making the diagnosis, an epidemiologic evaluation of the relation between analgesics and kidney failure would be biased.

Much of the work in pharmacoepidemiology today is conducted using health databases, which allow investigators to design studies from computerized files that include information on drug prescriptions, demographic factors, and health data from medical records or from claims data that deal with reimbursement. The Boston Collaborative Drug Surveillance Program was a pioneering effort in pharmacoepidemiology, starting with hospital-based interviews of inpatients using nurse monitors.[15] As the medical world gradually became more computerized, this work and that of other pharmacoepidemiologists evolved to use data that were already entered into computers as part of the record-keeping system, such as in some private prepaid health plans in the United States or governmental plans like that of the province of Saskatchewan in Canada. Pharmacoepidemiology is now an active field of research

---

When the disease definition includes an exposure

It is not only in the epidemiologic study of drugs that one encounters disease definitions that refer to exposures. If there is a clear understanding of a causal relation, it is a natural tendency to refine the definition of disease to reflect this insight. On the other hand, if the "insight" is only a presumption that a researcher would like to study, it is essential to apply disease definitions that are independent of the exposure. Following is a list of some examples of diseases defined on the basis of an exposure (most infectious diseases, such as syphilis and malaria, could also be included).

Analgesic nephropathy	Hypervitaminosis D
Asbestosis	Iron-deficiency anemia
Berylliosis	Motion sickness
Food poisoning	Protein-calorie malnutrition
Frostbite	Radiation sickness
Heat stroke	Silicosis

---

that has established itself as a separate specialty area with its own textbooks.[16,17]

Health-Outcomes Research

Health-outcomes research along with the related field of pharmacoeconomics are new research areas with lofty goals. Randomized trials and other medical research typically focus on a primary end point, such as survival or disease recurrence. Therapeutic evaluations based on narrowly defined end points have been subject to the criticism that they do not adequately take into account the overall quality of life that patients face, based on the combination of therapeutic outcomes and unintended effects that a given treatment produces. Furthermore, classic therapeutic research typically does not take into account the economic costs of different therapeutic options. The economic costs are borne either directly by the patient or insurers or indirectly by the government and, thus, society as a whole. In either case, there is strong motivation to find therapies that offer desirable results for patients at costs that are attractive to patients or society relative to the therapeutic alternatives. These are the goals that health-outcomes research and pharmacoeconomics address, using methods such as meta-analysis, cost-effectiveness analysis, decision analysis, and sensitivity analysis in addition to more traditional epidemiologic methods. The interested reader should consult Petitti[18] for a comprehensive overview of this dynamic research area.

Questions

1. Predictive value depends on disease prevalence, but sensitivity and specificity do not. What might cause the sensitivity and specificity of a test to vary from one population to another?
2. Suppose that you wished to conduct a prospective cohort study to evaluate the benefits of using prostate-specific antigen testing as a screening tool for prostate cancer. What outcome would most interest you? What biases would affect the study results? Would these biases also affect the results of a randomized trial?
3. Since everyone eventually dies, why would we not say that the case fatality rate among patients with any disease is 100%?
4. Under what conditions might one find that the baseline difference in a variable in a clinical trial is "statistically significant" but, nevertheless, not confounding? Under what conditions might we find that the baseline difference is not "statistically significant" but, nevertheless, confounding?
5. The Alzheimer's disease cooperative trial manifested confounding by score on the Mini-Mental State Examination. If the trial were repeated, would you expect that this same risk factor would be confounding again?
6. *Equipoise* is a state of genuine uncertainty as to which of two treatments is better. Ethicists consider equipoise to be an ethical requirement for conducting a randomized therapeutic trial: if the researcher is already of the view that one treatment is better than the other, then it would be unethical for that researcher to assign patients to the treatment that he or she believes is inferior. Under what conditions can equipoise be achieved in a placebo-controlled trial?

References

1. Catanzaro A, Perry, S, Clarridge, JE, et al: The role of clinical suspicion in evaluating a new diagnostic test for active tuberculosis. Results of a multicenter prospective trial. *JAMA* 2000;283:639–645.
2. Manos, MM, Kinney, WK, Hurley, LB, et al: Identifying women with cervical neoplasia: using human papillomavirus DNA testing for equivocal Papanicolaou results. *JAMA* 1999;281:1605–1610.
3. Cole, P, Morrison, AS: Basic issues in population screening for cancer. *J Natl Cancer Inst* 1980;64:1263–1272.
4. Chin, JE: *Control of Communicable Diseases Manual,* 17th ed. Washington, D.C.: American Public Health Association, 2000.
5. Rothman, KJ, Greenland, S: *Modern Epidemiology,* 2nd ed., Measures of disease frequency, p. 39. Philadelphia: Lippincott Williams & Wilkins, 1998.
6. Heart Outcomes Prevention Evaluation Study Investigators: Effects of an angiotensin-converting-enzyme inhibitor, ramipril, on cardiovascular events in high-risk patients. *N Engl J Med* 2000;342:145–153.

7. University Group Diabetes Program. A study of the effects of hypo-glycemic agents on vascular complications in patients with adult onset diabetes. *Diabetes* 1970;19(Suppl. 2):747–830.

8. Rothman, KJ: Epidemiologic methods in clinical trials. *Cancer* 1977; 39:1771–1775.

9. Friedman, LM, Furberg, CD, DeMets, DL: *Fundamentals of Clinical Trials,* 3rd ed., pp. 297–302. St. Louis: Mosby, 1996.

10. Sano, M, Ernesto, C, Thomas, RG, et al: A controlled trial of selegiline, α-tocopherol, or both as treatment for Alzheimer's disease. *N Engl J Med* 1997;336:1216–1222.

11. Pincus, MM: α-tocopherol and Alzheimer's disease. *N Engl J Med* 1997; 337:572.

12. Shapiro, AK, Shapiro, E: The placebo: is it much ado about nothing? In A. Harrington (Ed.) *The Placebo Effect. An Interdisciplinary Exploration,* p. 19. Cambridge, MA: Harvard University Press, 1997.

13. World Medical Association: Declaration of Helsinki. http://www.wma.net/e/policy/17-c—e.html.

14. Rothman KJ, Michels KB: The continuing unethical use of placebo controls. *N Engl J Med* 1994;331:394–398.

15. Allen, MD, Greenblatt, DJ: Role of nurse and pharmacist monitors in the Boston Collaborative Drug Surveillance Program. *Drug Intell Clin Pharm* 1975;9:648–654.

16. Hartzema, AG, Porta, MS, Tilson, HH: *Pharmacoepidemiology: An Introduction.* Cincinnati: Harvey Whitney Books, 1998.

17. Strom, BL: *Pharmacoepidemiology.* New York: John Wiley & Sons, 2000.

18. Petitti, DB: *Meta-Analysis, Decision Analysis and Cost-effectiveness Analysis.* New York: Oxford University Press, 2000.

Appendix p Values corresponding to values of the standard normal distribution (χ or Z) ranging from 0.00 to 3.99

χ Value in Tenths					χ Value in Hundredths					
	0.00	0.01	0.02	0.03	0.04	0.05	0.06	0.07	0.08	0.09
0.0	1.000000	0.992021	0.984043	0.976067	0.968093	0.960122	0.952156	0.944194	0.936237	0.928287
0.1	0.920344	0.912409	0.904483	0.896566	0.888660	0.880765	0.872881	0.865010	0.857152	0.849309
0.2	0.841480	0.833668	0.825871	0.818092	0.810330	0.802587	0.794864	0.787160	0.779477	0.771816
0.3	0.764177	0.756561	0.748968	0.741400	0.733856	0.726339	0.718847	0.711382	0.703945	0.696536
0.4	0.689156	0.681806	0.674485	0.667196	0.659937	0.652710	0.645516	0.638355	0.631227	0.624134
0.5	0.617075	0.610051	0.603063	0.596112	0.589197	0.582319	0.575479	0.568678	0.561914	0.555190
0.6	0.548506	0.541862	0.535258	0.528694	0.522172	0.515692	0.509254	0.502858	0.496504	0.490194
0.7	0.483927	0.477704	0.471525	0.465390	0.459300	0.453254	0.447254	0.441300	0.435391	0.429528
0.8	0.423711	0.417940	0.412216	0.406539	0.400908	0.395325	0.389789	0.384300	0.378859	0.373466
0.9	0.368120	0.362822	0.357572	0.352371	0.347217	0.342112	0.337055	0.332046	0.327086	0.322174
1.0	0.317310	0.312495	0.307728	0.303010	0.298340	0.293718	0.289144	0.284619	0.280142	0.275713
1.1	0.271332	0.266999	0.262714	0.258476	0.254286	0.250144	0.246048	0.242001	0.238000	0.234046
1.2	0.230139	0.226279	0.222465	0.218697	0.214975	0.211299	0.207669	0.204084	0.200545	0.197050
1.3	0.193601	0.190196	0.186835	0.183518	0.180245	0.177016	0.173830	0.170687	0.167586	0.164528
1.4	0.161513	0.158539	0.155607	0.152717	0.149867	0.147058	0.144290	0.141561	0.138873	0.136224
1.5	0.133614	0.131043	0.128511	0.126016	0.123560	0.121141	0.118760	0.116415	0.114106	0.111834
1.6	0.109598	0.107398	0.105232	0.103101	0.101005	0.098943	0.096914	0.094919	0.092957	0.091028
1.7	0.089131	0.087266	0.085432	0.083630	0.081859	0.080118	0.078407	0.076727	0.075076	0.073454

1.8	0.071860	0.070295	0.068759	0.067250	0.065768	0.064313	0.062885	0.061483	0.060108	0.058758
1.9	0.057433	0.056133	0.054858	0.053606	0.052379	0.051176	0.049995	0.048838	0.047703	0.046591
2.0	0.045500	0.044431	0.043383	0.042356	0.041350	0.040364	0.039398	0.038452	0.037525	0.036617
2.1	0.035728	0.034858	0.034006	0.033171	0.032354	0.031555	0.030772	0.030006	0.029257	0.028524
2.2	0.027806	0.027105	0.026418	0.025747	0.025090	0.024449	0.023821	0.023207	0.022607	0.022021
2.3	0.021448	0.020888	0.020340	0.019806	0.019283	0.018773	0.018274	0.017788	0.017312	0.016848
2.4	0.016395	0.015952	0.015520	0.015098	0.014687	0.014285	0.013893	0.013511	0.013138	0.012774
2.5	0.012419	0.012073	0.011735	0.011406	0.011085	0.010772	0.010467	0.010170	0.009880	0.009597
2.6	0.009322	0.009054	0.008793	0.008538	0.008290	0.008049	0.007814	0.007585	0.007362	0.007145
2.7	0.006934	0.006728	0.006528	0.006333	0.006144	0.005959	0.005780	0.005605	0.005436	0.005270
2.8	0.005110	0.004954	0.004802	0.004654	0.004511	0.004372	0.004236	0.004104	0.003976	0.003852
2.9	0.003731	0.003614	0.003500	0.003389	0.003282	0.003177	0.003076	0.002978	0.002882	0.002789
3.0	0.002699	0.002612	0.002527	0.002445	0.002365	0.002288	0.002213	0.002140	0.002070	0.002001
3.1	0.001935	0.001870	0.001808	0.001748	0.001689	0.001632	0.001577	0.001524	0.001472	0.001422
3.2	0.001374	0.001327	0.001282	0.001238	0.001195	0.001154	0.001114	0.001075	0.001038	0.001002
3.3	0.000966	0.000933	0.000900	0.000868	0.000837	0.000808	0.000779	0.000751	0.000724	0.000698
3.4	0.000674	0.000649	0.000626	0.000603	0.000581	0.000560	0.000540	0.000520	0.000501	0.000483
3.5	0.000465	0.000448	0.000431	0.000415	0.000400	0.000385	0.000370	0.000357	0.000343	0.000330
3.6	0.000318	0.000306	0.000294	0.000283	0.000272	0.000262	0.000252	0.000242	0.000233	0.000224
3.7	0.000215	0.000207	0.000199	0.000191	0.000184	0.000176	0.000170	0.000163	0.000156	0.000150
3.8	0.000144	0.000139	0.000133	0.000128	0.000123	0.000118	0.000113	0.000108	0.000104	0.000100
3.9	0.000096	0.000092	0.000088	0.000084	0.000081	0.000078	0.000074	0.000072	0.000068	0.000066

Index